A Woman Alone
Can Be
Contented

A WOMAN ALONE CAN BE CONTENTED

YOUR GUIDE TO SELF-FULFILMENT

LYNN UNDERWOOD

foulsham

LONDON • NEW YORK • TORONTO • SYDNEY

foulsham
The Publishing House, Bennetts Close, Cippenham, Slough,
Berks SL1 5AP, England.

ISBN: 0-572-02267-0

Typeset by ABM Typographics Ltd, Hull
Printed in Great Britain by
St. Edmundsbury Press, Bury St Edmunds, Suffolk

Contents

Introduction

*T*he idea for this book arose gradually – partly from my own experiences of living alone and partly from those of other women friends who live alone, particularly the elderly.

The idea for a book about living alone really crystallised when I was asked by a property magazine to write an article about viewing and choosing a home. I decided to approach it from the point of view of the single woman, of any age, and write about the careful selection of a home that was safe, secure and had all the amenities to hand. The article was a success and drew considerable response from the magazine's readers, many of whom were single and felt that most articles that dealt with this subject automatically assumed that home buyers were couples.

During the course of writing the article I researched the statistics on the number of people who live alone and was astonished. They make up a large percentage of the population and yet they do not appear to be catered for in any of the major bookshops. I found plenty of books and magazines about marriage and babies, some about retirement, some about teenagehood, but nothing about how to deal with the important stage in life experienced by practically everybody at one time or another – being alone. Of course, there were magazines catering for the 'swinging singles' – telling the readers how to have a great social life – but even they seemed to regard the single state as a temporary one and spent most of their time offering suggestions as to how one could share one's life.

It seemed to me that a positive tone was needed here. Many people enjoy living alone and there is nothing wrong with them. Many women find themselves living alone later in life and should be encouraged to enjoy it, but they are not. In the main, Victorian attitudes still prevail. Phrases like 'on the shelf' are still around while 'confirmed bachelor', 'spinster' 'career girl', 'widow' and 'widower' are used in the same vein as 'monk', 'nun' and 'hermit'.

I felt that this was wrong. Living alone can be a privilege, not a sentence. Your life is your own when you live alone. You do not have to bend to the demands and whims of others. You do not have to share your food, your wardrobe, your garden, or your time with anyone else. You may wish that you did. You may long for the right partner to come along. But, whether it is just for now or forever, you should resolve to enjoy your life alone and derive as much pleasure from it as you can.

With that philosophy in mind, I set about writing this book in the hope that it would give a fillip to a very neglected and underrated section of our society.

How to Have a Life, Not an Existence

When one lives alone, the world seems to be made up of couples but, in fact, it is not. In the United Kingdom, almost one third of the population lives alone; that is around twenty million people – hardly a minority group. What is more, owing to various factors, the number of people living alone is growing and the proportion of those who are women is growing even faster.

Women may live by themselves temporarily or permanently, by choice or by chance. They may start out their adult life living alone, or spend some of their middle years living alone, or end their days living alone. But what should be a happy and fulfilling experience all too often is not. This book is about deriving the best from that time of your life, whenever it occurs. It is about eliminating regrets, fears and anxieties and injecting a positive quality into time spent without other people.

That is not to say, however, that it is meant to praise living alone in preference to sharing your life. There is nothing wrong with living alone and hoping that one day you will share your life with another person. But such hopes should not overshadow any time alone to the extent that they lead to depression. No one should waste the potential for a good life by wishing that things were different.

Living alone does not have to mean solitary confinement. Friends and neighbours are not the prerogative of couples. Rather, it is the single woman who is in an ideal position to enjoy the perfect balance between a busy social life when she wants one and complete privacy when she doesn't. Being healthy and happy is the aim of the single woman as well as the married ones. She has an equal right not to dread going to bed alone, or dread waking up alone; there need be no loneliness on quiet Sundays.

There are many different reasons for being alone and different needs to be considered for the women who find themselves in that position. Many women find that they live alone through no design or plan. Life has just not provided them with a partner and they may not feel the lack of one.

Of course, a number of women start their period of being alone in some distress. Divorce, separation or bereavement mean that loneliness and grief play a large part in their lives for some time. But even if this is your situation, it is important to establish from the outset some degree of self-sufficiency to help you become stronger and happier eventually. The condition of happiness is, in the main, something we create ourselves by positive thought and action.

Some women make the choice to live on their own after they have tried various shared living arrangements and discovered that they prefer to be in control of their own lives and make their own rules. This is a perfectly good decision to make and will become a problem at a later stage only if they find that they have become too self-absorbed to be able to share their lives with another person.

Achieving total independence without loneliness or selfishness is a tricky business. Like everything in life that is worth having, it requires some effort and self-discipline. To create a quality of life that is admired by all your friends who do not live alone demands thought, planning, perseverance and a degree of practicality, although, in essence, all of this is determined by your will to live rather than merely exist.

LIFE IS WHAT YOU MAKE IT

Whatever the situation in which you find yourself living alone: whether your husband or lover has left you and the children have left home; whether your husband, lover or elderly parent has died; whether you are starting university or taking on a new job which is at the other end of the country – you must accept and make the very best of your new life. Each person has a different set of problems to face and overcome, but there are sources of help you can turn to so that you can cope with your circumstances and begin to think positively about your opportunities. In this book I have tried to list as many of these sources as possible, so that you can find support and information when you need them. I have also tried to cover the most common problems, doubts and fears that women living alone may experience. Of course, not all of this will be applicable or necessary to you. It is for you to select the information you want as and when you need it.

BEREAVED OR DIVORCED

If you are in this situation, the trauma of a bereavement or divorce is devastating. Women in these tragic circumstances have to come to terms with their sense of loss before they can come to terms with, and learn to enjoy, living alone.

A very large number of women who live alone do so not by choice, but as the result of the loss of a partner or family member. The first thing is to admit that, temporarily, you need support and help. Medication is not always the right resource in times of distress, but there are certain situations that are so terrible that you will need something to help you through the first few months. Visit your GP for advice but avoid turning to tranquillisers – no one benefits from making their life into a cotton wool ball. Many anti-depressants are non-addictive and your doctor will advise you on this. The fact is that you may need something to help you cope, sleep and carry on with your life. You may feel totally alone because you have relied on someone to do things with you and for you for some time. But you can do these things yourself. As for the things that you cannot do, you can ask a friend to help you or pay someone to do them for you. Hold on to that thought and try not to panic. You can do anything – eventually. You will be able to cope. Be patient with yourself because you will need to take time to heal yourself and recover your strength.

Thankfully, most women nowadays do not just sit back during marriage and let their partners pay all the bills, make all the decisions and run their lives. Most women participate fully in a partnership and therefore, if it should break down, are not left feeling totally helpless.

ORGANISATIONS TO HELP YOU

There are many groups, much literature and a great deal of help available for the bereaved and divorced – so much that to go into the subject in detail would require another book. However, I will mention here four of the largest and, I think, most useful groups whom you may wish to approach for advice and information. You will find local contact numbers for these organisations in your telephone book, and the addresses of the national organisations are listed at the back of this book.

Cruse

(The National Organisation for the Widowed and their Children)

CRUSE, and other organisations like it, provide support and a valuable shoulder to cry on when you do not know what to do. Apart from the support groups that CRUSE runs, it also provides a large range of literature about the problems of bereavement and provides practical help in dealing with paperwork and other matters that a bereaved woman may never have dealt with before.

Relate

(formerly The National Marriage Guidance Council)

RELATE recognised a long time ago that the fabric of society had changed, and one of the reasons for the organisation's change of name is that it now deals with personal relationship crises of any kind, whether you are married, single, heterosexual or homosexual. It also publishes some useful literature.

Age Concern

This group exists to help the elderly with all problems and, as a large proportion of their clients live alone, they are well-used to dealing with the difficulties of being single and lonely.

The Samaritans

The Samaritans are always there on the end of the phone to listen and help. Please do not think that only suicidal people ring up the Samaritans. Many of us sometimes need to talk through our day-to-day anxieties with someone other than a friend and the Samaritans are always glad to listen.

Financial Institutions

More and more, the financial institutions are beginning to recognise that those who are suddenly on their own, through bereavement, divorce or separation, are special customers who need help. Most banks, building societies and insurance companies will make suggestions on investing insurance money paid out on a death and give advice on money management generally. Remember, however, you should always consult several sources before making a decision about financial matters.

THE BREAKTHROUGH

Everyone who lives alone makes a breakthrough when they realise that living alone is not a prison sentence or a state to be endured. The real breakthrough happens when you feel confident about your status in life, your health, your financial situation etc. It does not necessarily mean happiness but it does mean confidence. You know that you can cope, that you have something to offer the world as an individual and you don't feel that you live alone because no one wants you. You may live alone because one person has said that he or she does not want to continue in a relationship with you, or you may live alone because the person you cared most about in the whole world has died, but you must remember that that one person does not represent the whole world. The breakthrough comes when you realise that living alone does not reflect on your value as a human being.

One day you will wake up (it may be a nice sunny Sunday morning) and you will luxuriate in the fact that you can do anything that you want to do – anything that takes your fancy – and there is no one else to consider.

A divorced friend of mine said that it took her about a year to reach the breakthrough. She said that she woke up one day and did not feel lost or depressed, did not wonder what she was going to do with herself and did not reach for the phone to try and summon up some company. She just sat over a leisurely breakfast and planned her day, and never looked back after that.

Another friend of mine, a woman who had spent most of her adult life looking after her elderly parents until they both died within a year of each other, came home from work one evening and suddenly realised that she could go to the cinema without worrying about anyone else. For ten months after her father's death she had unquestioningly taken the same train home, cooked a meal to be eaten at 7.30 in the evening (as she had always done when her parents were alive), watched television, made a cup of tea at 9.30 in the evening (as she had done when her parents were alive) and gone to bed. Her breakthrough was sudden and without apparent reason. She simply demolished the lifelong routine and began to build her own life.

The breakthrough may take the form of actually saying 'No' to a hectic social life. When I first left home and lived on my own, I gorged myself on an endless round of late-night parties and visits to new-found friends which lasted until the early hours of the morning. The exhilaration of not having to account for my movements to anyone went to my head. Then, after about three months, I had got it all out of my system, I suppose, and I actually turned down an invitation to a party in favour of staying in and washing some clothes! I had begun to desire some balance in my life and after that my socialising was toned down and my private moments stepped up.

The breakthrough comes when acceptance and relaxation come. It may be during your first week at work when a colleague asks you to join him or her in a group activity, such as a drink after work with friends. It may be that you receive praise for a piece of work well done, and suddenly you feel that you made the right decision to leave the family home and strike out on your own.

THE HERMIT COMPLEX

It is an ideal situation, when living alone, that you should enjoy your own company, but you should also balance this with forays into the outside world, otherwise solitude can become loneliness and seclusion can turn into a state of self-imprisonment. If you have no ready-made social life or circle of friends when you start your single lifestyle, then it requires more effort on your part. It is worth making the effort to involve yourself with other people but you do not necessarily have to share your home with them. Without social interaction we may begin to see life's problems out of proportion. It is too easy to lose control when one lives alone; the aim must always be to be 'alone but not lonely'. Social contact with others is a necessity and will be considered in greater depth in a later chapter.

ORGANISING YOURSELF

Being organised can take a great deal of worry out of a single life. For example, when I first lived alone, I used to be in a state of anxiety every time I left the house, for fear that I had forgotten something. I solved that problem by putting a notice on the inside of the front door which said:

HAVE YOU GOT YOUR KEYS?

HAVE YOU SWITCHED OFF THE GAS FIRE, THE ELECTRIC FIRE, THE OVEN, THE IRON, THE TV, THE RADIO ETC?

HAVE YOU LOCKED THE WINDOWS?

HAVE YOU GOT YOUR PURSE/HANDBAG/MEDICATION/ SEASON TICKET/ID CARD ETC?

It caused some mirth amongst my friends, but I noticed that several of them began to pin up similar notices in their own homes. I have also resorted to the pinned-up shopping list, this time in the kitchen. Whenever I think of something that is needed, I write it on my list. The tricky bit is remembering to take the list with me when I go shopping!

I now employ the list method for other things, planning my weekends for instance. I greatly enjoy sitting down on a Thursday evening to compile a list of all the pleasant (and unpleasant) things I have to do and then luxuriate in my sense of achievement on the following Sunday evening when every item on the list is ticked off. Keeping a diary is vital when you live alone because there is no one to remind you of your dental appointments or someone's birthday. I keep a pocket diary with me at all times and a calendar with spaces for writing on by the telephone. Then, at least once a week, I make sure that I bring both up to date.

Of course, today we have personal organisers, but I have never really been able to get on with these. The problem is remembering to consult them to find out what you should be remembering! I guess that bits of paper stuck on to walls works better for me – but you may be different. Use whatever suits you best to build some routine into your day-to-day life. There should be some routine in everyone's life, even if you are living alone. You need to establish some daily habits, no matter how tempting it is to lead an unfettered existence. This applies particularly if it is the first time you have lived on your own, otherwise you may find yourself persistently oversleeping, undereating or overspending.

Organisation does not mean martyrdom. Whether it

means buying an alarm clock, making packed lunches the night before, or ironing while you are watching television – method and routine, knowing what you have to do and the best way to do it, should make life more bearable. Be sensible in your plans though. There is no point in forcing yourself to do something after a hard day's work, for example.

Address books are vital, not simply for friends' addresses and phone numbers. Important names and addresses/phone numbers for any address book are:

DENTIST

DOCTOR

VET

BUILDER/HANDYMAN

PLUMBER

GARAGE

TAXI SERVICE

GAS COMPANY

ELECTRICITY COMPANY

INSURANCE COMPANIES

LOCAL POLICE STATION

LOCAL AUTHORITY (GENERAL NUMBER)

Keeping a filing system is an important means of organisation. The more things you acquire in life, especially when you buy a property, the more your paperwork accumulates. When you own a car you need to keep your driving licence, registration document, MOT certificate and the like somewhere where you can find them every time your car needs a new tax disc. I now keep all appliance handbooks and registration cards filed away so that I can diagnose faults in, say, the food mixer, without incurring expensive servicing.

Organisation means control, and control means peace of mind. Yes, it requires time and self-discipline, but since muddle, tension, anxiety and frustration do nothing to enhance the quality of your life, I am sure you will find that, in the end, it is worth the effort.

The Place Where You Live

This chapter is about your home and the decisions you may have to make about where you live. Whatever your circumstances, there is no doubt that your home surroundings are most important to the way you feel: making the right choices at the beginning can mean the difference between a home which gives you comfort and security or one which isolates you and becomes a financial burden.

WHETHER OR NOT TO MOVE

For many people who suddenly experience a change in circumstances, and for the disabled and elderly, the chance to move to a new home may seem like a good idea. The newly-divorced or widowed, in particular, may feel the need for a clean slate, a complete new start to their lives.

You may, of course, feel well settled in your present home, in which case this part of the book may not seem to apply to you. However, it is worth bearing in mind that your situation may change; keep an open mind and an eye on the future.

If you decide that you do want to move, think carefully

before you embark on such a course of action. Perhaps a retired person with no family ties can say 'Right, I'm selling up and moving to the Isle of Skye'. This may sound terrific in theory, but in practice will you really cope alone in a community where you know no one?

Beware of the 'retirement move syndrome' – many couples who have lived all their lives in suburbia retire and move to a quiet haven far from friends and family. Within two years the husband may die, leaving his widow alone and friendless without support in a community that she barely knows.

Understandably, people want to look forward to retirement, and for many people part of that dream is the rose-covered cottage or modern bungalow in the country or by the sea. However, not only are they moving away, but often they are also moving to a place totally unsuitable for elderly people. The south coast of England was revived by estate agents from a fading, genteel holiday coastline into a supposed retirement paradise, and yet winter by the sea (whatever the summer attractions) can be savage. Even a beautiful place such as Torquay will lose some of its appeal if a westerly wind is blowing the rain in your face. Cornwall and Devon have some of the steepest hills in the country – hardly suitable for someone who is elderly, and may well become frail. Equally, if you are divorced or bereaved, you should still bear in mind the pitfalls. You may, in the end, be happiest not moving.

THE CHOICE OF AREA

For those of us who are not free to live exactly where we want, because of various ties and commitments, picking a place to live is very, very important. The following is a checklist of the first three considerations which you should take into account before anything else:

- How mobile are you? Do you have a car or do you rely on public transport?

- Do you need to be near something e.g. schools, college, work, family, medical services?

- Do you want to be near something, such as friends, theatres, swimming pools, country parks, a bustling town?

Mobility, Needs and Wants

Your mobility to some extent governs the other two considerations. If you have a car then you have greater flexibility, but sometimes additional problems. For example, I live in a rural village that is prized because of its good connections with London. There are two stations within ten minutes' drive, from which travellers may be in London in under an hour. Neither of these stations is any use to me if my car is out of action, however, because I could not possibly walk to them. This happens to be all right for me because I do not commute every day to London, but if I did, then I would need to consider being closer to a station so that I was not totally reliant upon my car.

If you do not drive or you are approaching the age where you may have to give up your car, then you need to find an area where either everything you need is on your doorstep or the public transport service is very good and can take you efficiently wherever you need to go at the times you need to go.

Think carefully about things it is important for you to be near. You may want to be within an hour's journey of work or family. Think about what transport you would use and draw a circle on your map within which you can choose your area.

ASSESSING YOUR CHOSEN AREA

Once you have chosen the approximate area in which you want to live and the area that fits your first criteria of mobility, need and want, you must make a more detailed assessment:

What are the Local Amenities?

You will not always want to travel to the nearest town for your essentials. It helps if there is a little local parade of shops that covers everything – butcher, baker, grocer, greengrocer, and in particular a pharmacy, newsagents, doctor's surgery and post office. The last four are essential. No one wants to undertake a journey of any length if they are ill, much less to have a prescription filled out. A post office is invaluable because it can also act as a bank, not only during the week, but on Saturday mornings when normal banks are sometimes closed. It is always wise to have a source of money close at hand for emergencies, but not wise to keep it in the house. Of course, all banks now have cashcard points so that you can draw money out at any time, and most have more flexible opening hours nowadays and petrol stations and supermarkets will give you cash on a Switch card or other cash card. But it is sometimes useful to have a means of depositing money and this is where the post office can be invaluable.

If you work full-time, then it is useful to have a neighbourhood shop that opens early and closes late, so that you can get provisions before or after work.

Are the Emergency Services Convenient?

It is always comforting to have a hospital, fire station and police close at hand so that you know that they will not have far to come if you need them. However, I would not recommend having them next door, as I once did. There is little comfort in being woken up at three in the morning by sirens as police cars, fire engines or ambulances leave for an emergency.

What is the Local Weather Like?

This may sound a silly question, but it is more sensible than it sounds. Extreme weather conditions can easily affect your mobility and your health. The area where I live at present is bounded by two rivers and is quite close to the sea. What I did not realise when I moved here was that, in the winter, the fog rolls in so thickly that you cannot see your hand in front of your face.

There could be other peculiarities to the local weather. Homes near motorways or close to metropolitan traffic are often victims of 'summer smog', an acrid-smelling yellow haze which is caused by sunlight interacting with car exhaust fumes. Not a good idea if you suffer from respiratory problems.

A rural home may be idyllic but not if you suffer from bad hayfever and you are surrounded by farms growing oil-seed rape.

When you view that home tucked away down a winding country lane or up a hill, think about what it will be like in deepest winter when the frost starts to lay. Your car may not be able to cope!

Are There Any Local Problems?

People who buy or rent homes next to pubs, clubs or restaurants must be prepared for the consequences. Even the most refined restaurant is going to subject the surrounding properties to a certain amount of noise as people come and go – as is a large supermarket or a village hall.

Schools can be a problem as, today, almost every child is delivered to school by car and you suddenly find that at 8.30 in the morning and at 3.30 in the afternoon you cannot get your car out of your drive because the street is packed with vehicles unloading and loading children.

Being close to industrial estates, farms, or large shops can mean that you are subject to the constant rumbling of heavy transport going past your door.

You also need to find out whether there are any seasonal disturbances. Many people have viewed and bought a house in a quiet lane backing on to a field, only to find that, during the winter, the field becomes the frequently used local football pitch and every weekend is ruined by the shouting and screaming of supporters and players.

What is the Community Like Where You are Going?

Rurality is fine, but a village without a village hall suggests a lack of social life. The local library is the place to find lists of local societies and discover what is happening in the area. Social activities are important. Even if you do not have a social life when you settle in, you will eventually want something to do, and it is important to find out if your interests are catered for in the community.

Another factor in selecting a home and a potential social life is the predominant age of the community you have selected. Many new towns on the fringe of the affluent south east are so heavily populated by young married couples that they simply do not cater for retired people in any of their social activities. Similarly, you may be pushed to find an under-30s club in a known retirement area.

Are There Any Building Projects in Hand in Your Chosen Area?

Your solicitor will do a local search if you are buying a property but you may be renting, in which case, you will have to find out for yourself.

The local council offices will have details of any major plans that are being considered and you will have to go into the offices to look at them. If you do not do this research, then you may move into your home only to find that the road outside your flat is being widened into a motorway, or an incinerator plant is being built in the next village, or your uninterrupted view of woodland is to be spoiled by a new housing estate. Even smaller projects, such as a large extension to a neighbouring property, may affect you.

Is the Area Safe?

Women who live alone need to be especially secure from harm when coming and going to and from their home. Rural areas tend to be safer than urban areas as regards street crime but, perhaps, more vulnerable to burglaries and car thefts.

Look around the area. Is it well lit and policed? Would you be able to park your car off the road, in a garage or on your drive? If you have no car, would you have to cross lonely stretches of ground between your home and the bus stop or railway station? Would you have to pass potential trouble spots such as discos, pubs or clubs? Is the area prone to burglaries? Is there a Neighbourhood Watch Scheme? Go the the local library and read a few months' worth of back copies of the local newspaper. This should tell you what you need to know.

THE HOME ITSELF

When you are satisfied that the area you like is, in fact, all that you hoped it would be, then you can turn your attention to the actual property.

Rule number one, whether renting or buying, is never to take anything out of desperation – you will only regret it. Eventually, something better will turn up. It may take patience but it is a long-term decision so it is important to be fastidious about what sort of home you will be happy in.

Different women, naturally, have different requirements. A woman giving up her former marital home because of divorce or bereavement will probably be anxious not to sacrifice too much of the lifestyle she has enjoyed before. She will need space and comfort, perhaps a garden if she has always been used to one and enjoys gardening and, above all, she will need a property that gives her some self-esteem and security.

A young woman, in her first home, can probably accept a much lower standard, as long as it is dry and warm. The priorities will perhaps revolve more around it being convenient, easy to maintain and a good first base.

The disabled and frail elderly will, of course, have special requirements and will need to select a home that is manageable and is already, or can be, adapted to their specific needs.

Those women who are single and affluent will be looking for a home of some quality. Perhaps with their greater economic freedom they are most easily blinded by the options and may forget to take account of the special needs of women who live alone. Whatever the financial constraints or possibilities, it is important to remember your own specific needs.

Security

Whether you are renting or buying, your home must be safe. It does not matter how beautiful the décor, or how ravishing the garden, if it is not safe and secure you should not move in.

In an urban environment, basement flats are not advisable for the single dweller. The police report that over 40 per cent of burglaries of urban dwellings are break-ins to basement flats. They are easily accessible and hidden from view. They also have the disadvantage of being dark and prone to damp, and are seemingly tempting places for the general public to deposit litter – or worse – so do not hesitate to turn them down if you are offered any.

Flats with shared front entrances are not particularly desirable either, even if they do have entry phones fitted. It is too easy for a villain to con his way into an entrance hall by pressing any bell and claiming to be a delivery man. There is no efficient safeguard to ensure that you will not find such a person loitering in your entrance hall when you come home.

The best kind of flat is one above ground floor level that has its own entrance, providing that you do not gain access to your entrance up an unlit staircase or a long, dark walkway. The best option is a block of flats that has a resident caretaker who keeps a watchful eye over the block and is there to help in emergencies.

Do not be tempted to take a flat that is too high off the ground and requires the use of a lift. Not only will you have to have incredible stamina to cope with the stairs if the lift is out of action, but also lifts are like shared entrance halls – someone could loiter in a lift and present a danger. Also, lifts that are open to all and sundry seem to be readily vandalised or used as public toilets. Of course, there are elegant blocks of flats that have a full-time porter in the front reception or have electronic access only, but they are pricey.

Be realistic. Do not say 'I'm young and resilient, I can put up with a vandalised block of flats because it's a cheap place to live'. You could be putting your life, or at least your health, at risk for the sake of a few pounds. Even if you escape mugging or harassment, you may not escape the depression induced by your environment.

In urban or suburban environments, many of the flats on offer are in converted houses, which can be very good, or very bad. I have lived in a very good conversion and viewed some very bad ones. The same general rules apply to conversions as to purpose-built blocks: avoid basements and, if possible, choose one with well-lit, individual entrances. But when looking at conversions, you must be aware of the special kind of problems they may bring: look out for paper-thin dividing walls, bathrooms with no natural light or ventilation, and power points, or even doors, in awkward positions as a result of the subdivision of rooms.

If you are buying, then you will have a survey done, which should highlight any structural defects. Before you go to the expense of a professional survey, though, it is worth making a proper assessment yourself. You should also do this if you are renting – you are still proposing to enter into a contract with someone. Do not forget that, even if you are a potential council or housing association tenant, you still have the right to turn down unsuitable property or demand that certain repairs be carried out before you sign on the dotted line.

THE ART OF VIEWING

When you view a property use your nose, eyes and ears. Whether you intend to rent or buy, you need to make a detailed assessment of the property and whether it is suitable for you. Remember, of course, that you are viewing someone else's home and so be polite and considerate. But remember also that you are probably making one of the biggest investments of your life if you are buying, and whether you are buying or renting you are making a considerable commitment. Be assertive. You are quite within your rights to take a detailed look at the property and to visit it more than once if you are serious about it. Make sure that you see everything you want to see and receive answers to all your questions. Take a list to help you remember. Take a friend or adviser for support and encouragement if you need it.

What to Smell for ...

Firstly, note the smell when the present occupant opens the door. It is a little difficult to describe the smell of damp to those who have not encountered it, but it is a musty odour, rather like damp earth or leaves. Your nose may be assailed by all sorts of smells, of course. If the property has been lived in for a long time with old carpets that have never been shampooed, they can exude quite pungent odours.

There are other smells to be aware of, apart from damp. Gas, for a start. People can live for years with a small gas leak and never notice anything but always wonder why they are so tired. To a stranger, the smell may be rather more obvious. When you go to the bathroom, the smell of urine can mean that the toilet is leaking into the surrounding floorboards – an expensive business to correct.

Try not to view a property when the present occupant is likely to be cooking a meal because that will effectively swamp all other smells. However, do take note if there is a lingering odour of cooked food at other times. This may mean that the ventilation in the flat is inadequate – the kitchen may need to be fitted with an extractor fan, for example.

If there is a powerful smell of dogs or cats, this in itself may not be a problem for you after the present occupant and pets have left. But a very strong smell should make you wary. Pets can harbour fleas, which love fitted carpets, and if the owner is not aware of or does not deal with the infestation, you may be left to deal with it when you move in.

Do not be seduced by good smells either. It is a well-known ploy for owner-occupiers who are trying to sell their properties to have fresh coffee brewing or bread or cakes baking. Such mouthwatering smells can only serve to overcome your better judgement!

What to Look for ...

Firstly look at the layout of a flat. Some conversions that were done a long time ago would not pass today's stringent building regulations.

For example, if a flat has only one entrance/exit and it is above ground floor level, it should have a fire escape or some means of escape over a balcony or a roof. Seventy per cent of all home fires start in the kitchen, so a converted flat that has a kitchen next to the front door – the main entrance/exit – is dangerous. It means that you could be trapped in the flat if a fire breaks out.

There are also strict rulings on bathrooms and separate lavatories. If these rooms have no window in an outside wall, then an electric ventilation unit must be installed.

You can obtain information about building regulations from your local council planning department.

Does the living room get plenty of light? Most of your

activities will be in here – sewing, reading, watching television, entertaining and so on – and you should not have to have artificial light on all the time to do them.

If you can possibly afford it, opt for more than one bedroom. This gives you so much more flexibility to have people to stay, to rent out a room if you become hard up or to simply move into one room yourself while you decorate the other. If you are buying a property, you should always try and maximize your resale potential. Two-bedroomed flats can be bought by a variety of people. One-bedroomed flats are restricted to single purchasers, in the main.

Think of flexibility again in the bathroom. A separate toilet is ideal because, if you do have people to stay or you take in a lodger temporarily, it is less of a problem if one wants to go to the toilet while the other is having a bath or shower. Similarly, bathrooms that can only be reached by going through one of the bedrooms are not a good idea.

Look at the number and size of the rooms and be realistic. Can you fit everything you have into the space, and can you do all the activities you need in such space? You may need somewhere to study or to do your hobby. You may entertain a lot and need a separate dining room.

If you are disabled in any way (even if it is only a minor disability, it could become worse as you get older) then you must view a property from the point of view of your ease of movement. Are the doorways wide enough for a wheelchair? Can you go easily from one room to another? Is the floor level throughout or are there steps up and down to various rooms? If you can manage to live in a house now but may need to install a chair lift on the stairs when you get older, are the stairs straight and able to take such a fitment?

Check that the worktops in the kitchen are at the right height for you. Can the walls withstand the installation of special equipment such as bed-hoists or bath rails? If you are disabled, take a specialist adviser along with you to view a property to consider any problems in structural adaptation. If you get to the point of seriously considering a particular property, then your local Social Services department should be able to advise you about whether certain adaptations can be made and where. Also they should be able to give advice on whether you will get assistance with the cost of repairs that are needed.

Still relying on your eyes, look at the window frames. Are they rotting and peeling? Are the sash cords intact? Do the windows open and close easily? Look at the putty that secures the glass in place. It may be old and cracked and bits may have fallen out. Panes of glass may be cracked. All these will have to be replaced or you will feel draughts. Look at doors and close them. Are they hanging well, do they close properly? Are there large gaps at the top and the bottom of the doors? If so, there will be more draughts.

Look at taps. Are they dripping? Is the mastic around the base of the taps worn away?

Look at the front door. From the point of view of security you do not want a door that is all glass, neither do you want a hollow plywood-type door that is easily kicked in. A solid door that has good secure locks – preferably two, a Yale lock and a deadlock – and in which you can install a viewer, which will enable you to verify the identity of callers before you open the door, is an important feature.

Look at the ceiling. Sometimes it is difficult to tell whether ceilings are badly cracked because people cover them up with ceiling paper, tiles or Artex.

It's the same with walls. You can look for damp patches, though, particularly on outside walls. There will be telling changes in the colour of the wallpaper or paint surface inside. Be assertive when you are viewing a property. Move sofas away from the walls and look carefully.

Look at the electrical points. If they appear new, then the electrical wiring is possibly up to scratch, since no professional electrician would install new power points without checking the wiring first. Beware of anything that looks like a do-it-yourself job – crooked power points for example. Are there enough power points, particularly in the kitchen? Does the property have gas and electricity? If so, where are the meters? Do you have easy access to the stopcock that turns off the water? This is most important in an emergency, and so its position should be remembered and it should never be boarded up.

Look at the floors. Are they even or do they slope in some rooms? Old properties can be subject to settlement. If it is possible, take up the carpet and look at some of the floorboards. You should see what condition they are in, if only to see whether you could, if you wished, take up the carpets and have stripped and polished floors.

What to Listen for ...

Are the walls solid or can you hear the neighbours clearly through them? It is a good idea, particularly with flats, to view them at times when you know all the residents will be at home, to see if you can hear the television upstairs or the stereo downstairs. Do the floorboards creak? Can you hear the upstairs neighbour walking across the floor? Can you hear the traffic in the busy road outside? Can you hear other neighbourhood noises which you will find irritating? For example, if you are going to be home all day and there is a school nearby, will it drive you mad to hear the playground noises at breaks and lunchtimes? Try viewing a property near a hospital on a Saturday night and see if the evening is constantly interrupted by ambulance sirens. It may be nice to live near a church but do they have regular bell-ringing practice and are the bells constantly ringing on Saturdays for weddings? Listen, on a weekend, for the noise of DIY enthusiast neighbours. There is nothing quite as irritating as someone who comes home from work and gets out an electric drill every night. If you want peace and quiet, then you probably do not want to move into a property where you are surrounded by young families with crying babies and noisy older children. Barking dogs are not a problem if they only bark at intruders. They are a form of security for you as well as your neighbour but do remember that some dogs bark incessantly.

SOME EXTRA POINTS ...

The biggest expense of any house, and its most important facet, is the roof. At first glance, you will only be able to tell whether the roof is old or new. Look more closely for moss growing on tiles, cracked tiles and damaged chimney stacks. You will need a surveyor, or a friend in the building trade, to inspect the loft and check whether all is dry and whether the timbers supporting the roof are sound. If there is no loft because it has been converted into a bedroom, look for the tell-tale signs of damp, or listen, on a windy day, for the noise of wind rushing through the eaves. It is common practice for house sellers to furnish a timber or roof survey if they have had the roof or timbers repaired or treated in any way. Be sure to ask if such a thing exists.

The garden or gardens, front and back, also need to be considered carefully. Please be realistic about them. You will be living there on your own and may be out a lot, either at work or socially, during the week. Even if you love gardening, you should only take on a garden that you can easily manage. If you are elderly, a small garden may provide the pleasure you gain from gardening, without too much hard work. Remember your personal security when viewing front gardens. Without wishing to be alarmist, a garden with lots of high foliage gives a burglar or mugger lots of cover. Look for a very open front garden which gives the front of your house some clear visibility. Alternatively, resolve to chop down the existing jungle when you decide to take up residence. The only thing that should be able to hide in your front garden is a garden gnome.

Never buy or rent a house with a back garden that backs on to a public footpath or alleyway, or a house that has a public path running down the side of the garden. These are security risks. Also, children are likely to play ball against your side wall and you may find yourself picking out of your garden litter which has been thrown over the fence. Unfortunately, front and side gardens in urban areas can be magnets for litter louts.

If the garden does not already have them, then you might like to erect fences or walls that are high enough to deter intruders and give you some privacy. If the neighbours think that you are being anti-social, you can always make the excuse that you have a passion for climbing plants. Bushes with thorns and spikes, like holly, are excellent to plant inside fences to deter intruders. If you feel this is necessary, however, remember the cost before deciding that it is essential.

Before you commit yourself to your chosen home, make sure that you know all about the boundaries of your property, any rights of way that exist, such as neighbours having access over your gardens and which fences you have to maintain.

Your solicitor, during the course of making enquiries about the home you are going to buy, may fail to uncover a right of way because it may not be registered, and the present occupant of the property may not be aware that there is a legal right. The present occupant may say 'Oh well, I let old Mrs Smith walk through my garden and down the sideway when she needs to' and regard it as no more than a neighbour's agreement. However, if this practice has persisted for more than 12 years it will have become what is known as a prescriptive right of way, which you will inherit and be unable to change. The tell-tale signs are gaps in the fence between you and your potential neighbours, or even gates and doors.

Garages are lovely things to have, if they are attached to your house, but can be a source of grief if they are part of a block that is situated away from the property. You are liable to find that every time you go to use your car one of any number of people has parked in front of your garage and you cannot get your car out. Also, a remote block of garages can be a magnet to car thieves, if it is not visible from the houses. Unlit garage blocks can also be a personal security hazard if you have to park and walk some distance to your house at night.

I mentioned staircases earlier in the chapter, with a view to installing stair lifts, but there are other points to consider as well. For example, if the staircases are very twisting, such as spiral staircases, can you get furniture upstairs? You may have to remove the windows and winch furniture up or you may even have to build flat-pack furniture *in situ*.

If you are renting or buying a flat, or moving into sheltered accommodation, what are the service charges? A recent development in the property market has been the creation of a large number of sheltered accommodation units, both rented and private. This is an excellent idea for the elderly or the housebound as it provides independent, secure accommodation with fitted alarms linked up to a 24-hour warden service. However, some elderly people have bought such accomodation without properly investigating all the costs involved. There is often a very high service charge to pay for all the administration, the maintenance service – such as cleaning of communal areas, gardening and repairs – and, of course, the wardens. Many blocks of flats, for all ages, have service charges attached, so make sure that you know all about them, down to the last penny, before committing yourself.

Also, if you are disabled or elderly but prefer not to live in sheltered accommodation, you may need to organise, through your local Social Services department, a 'care package' which will enable you to live an independent life in your chosen home.

Care packages, which are now provided by independent agencies, can range from just a little house cleaning a couple of times a week to having 24-hour care – and you will have to pay for those services. Care in the community is not free any more.

There is also something called ground rent, which is attached to leasehold flats. The person who owns the entire building, whether it is a converted house or purpose-built block, sells the flats on long leases and charges the owners of the flats an annual ground rent. Out of this, the owner of the whole building supposedly takes some responsibility for certain external repairs to the fabric of the building. When I lived in South London, unscrupulous property developers were buying up the freeholds of converted houses at auctions and raising the ground rents to astronomical figures in order to force people to sell their flats back to them. Recently, there has been a movement by leasehold flat owners to band together, form a management company and buy up their own freeholds, thus ensuring that their ground rents remain low.

Active residents' and tenants' committees in your block, estate or area are a good sign. They give you a point of contact with neighbours and usually mean that your environment is afforded some degree of protection by the efforts of these people.

Finally, we come to the bugbear of many residents – rubbish collection. Now that we have the practice of dustmen only collecting plastic bags of rubbish that you have to place outside your residence, you have to be sure that you are capable of doing just that. If you are elderly or disabled and the rubbish has to be taken down to the end of a long driveway, can you cope? Some purpose-built blocks fortunately have rubbish chutes on each landing which means that you can dispose of your rubbish in small quantities daily, down to a large bin. If your flats do not have this facility, however, where do you store all the rubbish as it accumulates? This is a problem that is easily overlooked when viewing a property.

Working from Home

If you intend to work as well as live in your home you have to make sure that your type of work does not infringe any conditions in your tenancy, your insurance or any local by-laws. For example, you may make craft items at home, either for yourself or an employer, that involves the use of flammable materials. If you have a fire and the insurance company find out that you have been operating in this way, they will almost certainly refuse to pay out unless they knew about the risks beforehand and included it in their premiums.

Tenancy agreements may prohibit the operation of certain businesses from home, such as anything hazardous or noisy. This might include the operation of industrial sewing machines, or other noisy machinery. Council tenancies have quite strict clauses about operating any business from a council property.

The council and the neighbours might take a dim view of you operating from home a business which is noisy, messy or affects parking in the street. You might, for example, have constant deliveries to your home by lorries which irritate the neighbours and cause traffic congestion. You might do something as innocent as give piano lessons at home but the noise pollution regulations are so stringent nowadays that unless your home is properly soundproofed you could find an environmental health inspector turning up as a result of neighbours' complaints. Do check with your local council before you start any business from home.

Renting a Property

All the information in this section has been supplied by the Department of the Environment and the Welsh Office. Laws may differ slightly in Scotland.

If you have never rented a property before, it is worth knowing what you should expect from the contract that you are undertaking. Whether you are renting privately, from a housing association or from a council, you should have a proper tenancy agreement that gives rules of occupation which list what you can and cannot do, such as keep pets or alter the structure of the property. The agreement should also outline the landlord's obligations, such as repairs. You must also have a rent book, if you pay rent weekly, as proof of your financial transactions. You should receive receipts for all payments made which are not weekly.

Types of Tenancy

There are several types of tenancy:

Regulated tenancies: These can either be protected or statutory. The difference is that a protected tenant has security by virtue of his or her contract with the landlord; a statutory tenant has security by virtue of the protection given by the Rent Acts.

Shorthold tenancies: A new type of regulated tenancy introduced in 1981, these are tenancies that are for a fixed period of one to five years, after which the landlord has a guaranteed right to repossess the property. Other situations where a landlord has a guaranteed right of repossession are: lettings by temporarily absent owner-occupiers; lettings of retirement homes (a letting that enables people to let a home to which they intend ultimately to retire) and lettings by servicemen.

I should mention here the recent practice by building societies and other financial institutions of buying the homes of elderly owner-occupiers and allowing them to live in the property for the rest of their lives. In recent years it has become an excellent way of releasing the capital tied up in a home if the owner-occupier has no desire to leave the property to relatives after death. Financial institutions have developed the practice of buying these homes (at less than the market value, it has to be pointed out) and entering into a tenancy agreement which allows the former owner to reside in the property until they die or need to move (to live either with family or in a nursing home). At this time the property reverts to the lender and is theirs to sell. This option is only available for those over retirement age and, in some cases, older.

Restricted contracts: This is the legal term for lettings where the landlord and tenant live in the same house. Tenants of resident landlords do not normally have long-term security of tenure, and such lettings are not subject to the fair rent system.

Assured tenancies: These are due to be phased out over the next year, so you will not be able to negotiate a tenancy of this kind.

Local authority tenancies: Local authority and housing association tenants have certain rights that are laid down by government:

§ The right to buy their home (after a certain period of tenancy and subject to meeting financial criteria).

§ Security of tenure, subject to their landlord being able to regain possession of the property on certain defined grounds, such as not paying their rent.

§ The right of a widow, widower or resident member of their family to succeed to the tenancy on the tenant's death.

§ The right to exchange their home.

§ The right to take in lodgers.

§ The right to sub-let part of their home (as long as they do not change the use, by sub-letting to a business concern for example).

§ The right to repair their home.

§ The right to information about their legal rights and obligations and those of the landlord.

§ The right to be consulted about matters affecting their tenancy.

§ Certain rights about communal heating charges.

Private tenants also have certain rights:

§ The right to apply to a rent tribunal to fix a fair rent.

§ The right, if they pay a service charge, to obtain a summary of the costs on which their service charge is calculated and to inspect the accounts and receipts on which the summary is based.

§ The right to ask a court to fix the amount that they

have to pay for services and works, on the grounds that these have not been provided to a reasonable standard at a reasonable cost.

๕ The right to ask a court to limit to what is reasonable the amount of any advance payments their lease requires them to make against a service charge.

๕ The right for a tenants' association to be officially recognised.

๕ The right to a valid notice to quit, in writing, served at least four weeks before the tenancy is due to expire, which must also contain certain prescribed information about tenants' rights.

There are two final points of law that you should be aware of: firstly, when a tenant's right to occupy comes to an end, the tenant cannot be made to leave against his or her will, except by a court order. Eviction without a court order is a criminal offence

Secondly, if the tenancy was granted for less than seven years, the landlord is, by law, responsible for the repair of the structure and exterior of the dwelling and for keeping in repair and proper working order any basins, sinks, baths, and other sanitary installations, and any installations for supplying gas, water, electricity, for heating water, and for space heating

Buying a Home

Buying a property is an exercise in frustration – always. From the time you fall in love with a property to the time you move in, you can count on it taking an average of three to four months. It can take much longer if you are selling as well as buying, for you are then involved in a dreaded thing called 'a chain', which only moves at the pace of the slowest buyer or seller, that is if it does not disintegrate altogether along the way and put you back to square one.

When you find a place that is satisfactory, though, the first thing to do is make an offer for it to the vendor's estate agent. This does not have to be at the advertised price. If you genuinely think that the property is worth less than the asking price, then make a lower offer. Most vendors allow for a margin of negotiation anyway. If your offer is acceptable, then you proceed by applying for a mortgage (see below) and informing your appointed solicitor or conveyancing agent of the details of the purchase so that he can make formal overtures to the vendor's solicitor.

Mortgages

Most people buy a home with the help of a mortgage via a building society, bank, insurance company, house builder or local authority. However, if you are in the position of selling a larger property, which is paid for, and buying a smaller one, then you may not have to raise finance. It used to be the case that one had to find a property that one wanted to buy and then apply for a mortgage, but some organisations will now provide a mortgage guarantee document, that is to say, an assurance of the amount of money that they will lend you, subject to the chosen property being suitable, before you start looking for a property.

Either way, the amount of money you can borrow will be based, if you work, upon a multiple of your earnings –

usually two and a half to three times the value of your gross earnings per year. For example, if you earn £10,000 per year, then you may be able to get a mortgage of £30,000. The percentage of the purchase price that is advanced may depend upon the age of the property. Most organisations do not lend 100 per cent of the purchase price on old properties, and the amount of money they will eventually advance you depends upon the recommendations of their surveyor. If he says that the property is not worth the asking price, then the lender will only offer you the amount recommended by the surveyor.

Shop around for a mortgage. All of the building societies, at the time of going to press, are offering special deals to first-time buyers and those who will re-mortgage with them. In some cases they are even offering to give cash back or pay survey fees, solicitors' fees or removal expenses. Many new housebuilders are even offering to buy your old property so that you do not get caught in a chain. You can choose between variable and fixed rate mortgages and there is a whole range of other options. If you do not feel confident in making decisions without advice, contact an independent mortgage adviser to guide you through the maze and help explain all the various factors involved.

Surveys

There are usually two types of surveys: a valuation survey and a more in-depth one. At first the valuation survey will be all you need. You may have to pay for it or it may be provided by the mortgage lender. It will consist of about two sides of an A4 sheet, giving you only very basic details about the property unless there are, on cursory inspection by the surveyor, some very obvious defects, such as a roof in a bad state of repair or obvious damp penetration on walls. The purpose of this survey is simply to recommend to the lender the true value of the property. Based upon this assessment the lender will offer you a mortgage, but it may be conditional upon certain repairs being carried out.

This is where the first problems may occur. If the surveyor states that the property is most definitely not worth the asking price, you have four options: abandon the property and look elsewhere; find the cash to supplement the shortfall in the mortgage offered; go to another building society and hope that another surveyor will not make the same judgement; or go to your vendor's estate agent, explain the situation and hope that the vendor will drop the price. Whichever way you choose, you will not get the money back that you have spent on the valuation survey. Therefore, it is best to not throw further money at your house-buying process and, if your vendor will not drop the price sufficiently, then look at another property. Unfortunately, every property that takes your fancy will entail paying for another survey. That is why it is always best to examine a property thoroughly or take a friend with you who will help you to spot potential problems in the property before you make an initial offer.

Once you decide to go ahead, it can be a good idea to commission an in-depth survey which will go into more detail on the state of the property. A survey like this will cost several hundred pounds but it should uncover any problems or potential problems and will highlight greater detail, such as decorative repairs, which may not affect the price of the property but which still need attention. A word of caution about buying property at auctions: it is true that you can pick up some bargains at property auctions but only if you know what you are doing and what your potential cash outlay could be. Properties that go in auctions are usually 'problem' properties, i.e. they may be in great need of renovation (you may be able to get grants for installing bathrooms, plumbing and rewiring), or they have sitting tenants, or they are difficult to sell in other ways. It is rare to be able to get a mortgage for such properties, so you need to have cash in hand. And, once your bid at an auction has been accepted by the auctioneer, it is considered legally binding – you cannot change your mind – and you will be expected to pay a percentage of the purchase price immediately, with the rest to follow within a specified timespan of rarely more than a few weeks.

Buying at auction is not something for the novice home owner.

Conveyancing

Assuming you are buying a conventional property and your survey is fine, then your solicitor or conveyancing agent will make pre-contract enquiries, which means that the vendor's solicitors will have to answer various questions about boundaries, fences, drains etc. A local search will be instituted, which means that the person acting on your behalf will apply to the local authority for any information regarding roadworks, planning matters, footpaths, or anything else that might affect your property and its environs. He will also apply to the Land Registry for copy title deeds of the property and a potted history of various ownerships. All this activity will take a month or more. In some areas local authorities are so understaffed and overworked that searches can take much longer. I have heard of the practice of solicitors buying local searches from the vendor's solicitors but I do not know whether the practice is widespread.

This is the time to make sure you get all possible information – you don't want any nasty suprises later on. Talk to the neighbours, talk to local people, find out what the local grapevine is saying about the area. Read some back issues of local newspapers. Tell your solicitors if you suspect that there might be a right of way 'agreement' between neighbours that would not be written down or if you have heard a rumour about a development proposal that could blight the area.

Deposits

If the pre-contract enquiries and the local search are satisfactory, then you can proceed to sign the contract and pay a deposit. This is where you may have another problem, particularly if you are a first-time buyer, because the deposit payable is usually five per cent of the total value of the property, sometimes ten per cent. That means that you have to find, for example, £2,000 to £4,000 in ready money as a deposit on a £40,000 house. The organisation lending you the money will not advance this to you, and so you have to find it from somewhere else – either your savings or a short-term loan.

Completing the Deal

The completion date (i.e. when you actually move in and the money for the property is handed over) is usually 28 days after the exchange of signed contracts and deposits. So you will be without your deposit money for a month at least. Of course, it will be returned to you by the solicitor, less all the expenses incurred in conveyancing when you move house.

If you are selling as well as buying, your solicitor will not allow you to use your purchaser's deposit for your own deposit to your vendor.

If you are selling as well as buying, then the whole business is doubled up – you have to answer pre-contract enquiries from your purchaser's solicitor, as well as obtaining them from your vendor. Your purchaser will have a survey done and institute a local search on your property. All of this adds to the time involved in the process and also, of course, adds to the fees.

Fees and Costs

The fees payable for the whole process are as follows:

Arrangement fee: Some lending organisations charge a mortgage arrangement fee, which can vary from a few pounds to nearer £100.

Survey fees: Usually this is a fixed sum which, at the time of writing, seems to average around £150. Prices for a structural survey start at around £300 and an average figure would be £500–600.

Solicitor's/conveyancing agent's fees: These vary, since the introduction of licensed conveyancers and new laws which has allowed solicitors to advertise has made the whole marketplace more competitive. Many are offering fixed rates for simple conveyancing, such as a purchase by a first-time buyer. Fees will average several hundred pounds.

Stamp duty: This is payable on all properties valued at over £60,000 and is calculated at a fixed rate of one per cent. Therefore the stamp duty on a house worth £70,000 is £700. Do make sure that any monies paid for fixtures and fittings are excluded from the registered purchase price, otherwise you will pay stamp duty on them.

Land Registry fees: This varies according to the purchase price; it starts at £40, but rises sharply according to house price.

Search fees: This varies according to the local authority involved but it is usually about £50.

Deposit: This is usually a standard ten per cent of the purchase price in contracts but in practice is sometimes agreed at five per cent.

Estate agent's commission: This is only applicable if you are selling a property through an estate agent and is usually between one and two per cent of the purchase price. In real terms it can be a large sum to pay (£700–£1,400 plus VAT on a £70,000 sale) so think carefully when you budget for a move.

Bridging loans: If you are selling a house and buying another one, you may find yourself in a position where you have to wait for your purchaser to complete, whereas your new home is ready and must be paid for. You will therefore be put in the position of paying two mortgages at the same time for a short period.

Unless you have enough spare cash to do this, you will have to take out a bridging loan. Interest rates on such loans vary.

Removal costs: Shop around for a reasonable estimate, or hire a van and the services of some friends and do it yourself. It is much cheaper and definitely worthwhile if you are young, strong and don't have much heavy furniture. Otherwise it is a false economy, as removal men can move you quickly and expertly without any hassle or danger of doing themselves an injury in the process.

ORGANISING THE MOVE

Once you have rented or bought your home, and you have fixed a date for your occupation, it is time to sort out the essential services – gas, electricity, water and telephone. You will need to telephone the various local offices (local, that is, to the place where you are going to live) and make sure that a telephone will be laid on, the gas and electricity meters will be read and that all the services will be connected and functioning when you arrive on the day.

This can be difficult. If you have, for example, never been a telephone subscriber before (this applies even if you have had the use of a telephone but it was not in your name) you will have to pay a new subscriber charge plus a connection charge. If you want to organise your energy bills to be paid monthly instead of quarterly, tell the gas and electricity companies at this stage. If you need to have your gas fire or cooker connected when you arrive at your new place, make sure that you tell the gas company that you need someone there on the day. It may, in fact, be better to organise it all for the day after you move, because being certain that everything will run according to plan on the day of the move is almost impossible. It is better to do without your cooker overnight and go and buy fish and chips.

If you are moving from a place other than a shared home for which you had no responsibilities, you will need to cancel the milk and newspapers for ever, and organise new deliveries at your new address. This will necessitate a visit to the local newsagent for the papers and you will have either to ask your new next door neighbour if he or she can give a note to the milkman for you, or contact the local dairy yourself.

You will also find it helpful to have your post redirected. This is done by going to your local post office, filling in a form and paying a small fee – the amount depends on how long you want the post redirected but most people find that three months is adequate. Your change of address is important to all your friends and relatives and all those people who usually send you bills and communications – like the bank, building society, post office, insurance company etc., and you should notify them straight away.

Packing

If you are using a removal firm, ask them to provide tea-chests/packing cases for all the small items. You can pack them yourself or the removal firm will do them for you. If you are carrying out the move yourself, with the help of some friends, then do not use tea-chests, they are too heavy.

Start scouring your local supermarkets and off-licences for strong cardboard boxes. Select the ones that have held bottles, because they will be stapled at the bottom and are much stronger. Also look for ones that have carrying slots at either side as they are much easier to manage. Save newspapers for wrapping china.

Label all the boxes with the contents and make an inventory of every box. This serves several purposes: it will identify your belongings from those of other people's that may also be in the removal van; it will help you and your friends, or the removal men, to put the boxes in the right rooms at the other end. And if the box is labelled 'kitchen crockery' this will enable you to lay your hands quickly on the teapot when it is all over and you are gasping for a cuppa!

Sort out any booklets or manuals that pertain to the heating system or any other fixture that you are leaving behind. Write out a list of local phone numbers and any instructions that the next occupants of your home will find invaluable – like how to open that funny cupboard in the second bedroom that always sticks. Ask the occupants of your new home if they would please do the same thing for you before you move in. Start running down the food in the fridge and freezer in advance, so that they can be switched off and cleaned a couple of days before you move. Clear out your food cupboard and throw away everything that will not travel well, such as leaky, crushable or carbonated goods. Make a list of what essential food you will need for the first day in your new home and go shopping the day before you move.

Clear out all your possessions and be ruthless. Now is the time to take rubbish to the dump and to give things away to charity shops and jumble sales. There is no point in taking all your useless junk with you. Also, clear up the garden. You are not supposed to leave refuse behind you for the next occupants to cope with, although you can leave it bagged up outside the door for the dustmen to take later.

If you are leaving the area, do not forget to pick up any clothes that are at the cleaners, or shoes, clocks, or any other items that are away being mended. Return all library books. You will also need to withdraw sufficient cash from the bank to pay for the removal. It is common practice to tip the people who have done the removal work.

On the day of the removal, board pets with friends for the day. It is too upsetting for them and, anyway, dogs and cats will get under your feet. Pack everything except some cleaning materials and the vacuum cleaner, so that you can clean all the corners and places where hidden dirt is revealed once the furniture is removed. It is also not a bad idea to pack the kettle, a jar of coffee, a vacuum flask of milk and some mugs.

You may want to make the nice gesture, which was made to me when I first moved into a flat and which I have repeated myself whenever I have moved, of leaving a plant or a box of chocolates and a note wishing the next occupants a happy life in your former home.

You will need to make arrangements for handing over and/or collecting all the keys to the properties on the day of the removal.

Money – Do You Have Enough?

When you live alone money assumes a greater importance than if you share your life with someone. Why? You have no family to feed and clothe, you should have less of a problem. But the old saying 'a problem shared is a problem halved' is very true. Two people can cope with money worries better than one. You only have yourself to fall back on, unless, of course, you count a friendly bank manager who might lend you some money, or a friend or relative who might do the same. But borrowing money that you are going to have difficulty paying back only adds to your anxieties. So try to avoid it.

The way to manage money is firstly to assess what you have coming in and what you have to pay out. Budgeting is an instant turn-off to many people. Organising your financial well-being, however, should prove more relaxing in the long run. To be fair to yourself you should be certain that you are bringing in as much money as possible.

How Much is Coming In? (And Going Out)

One of the first things you should check – assuming that you have a job – is that your tax code is correct and that you are receiving all the allowances, grants and benefits you may be able to claim. We are not talking about charity here, we are talking about money that you are entitled to, that you have earned through the taxes you have paid. There are charitable awards which you may wish to ask for too, but I shall come to them later in this chapter.

Income Tax

Let us look at your tax code first. When you fill in your Income Tax Return, you must declare all your sources of income and the Inspector of Taxes will ignore them or assess tax as necessary. More importantly, perhaps, he (or she) may even give you a tax rebate if you have overpaid somehow. It is therefore vitally important that you fill in the Return correctly in order to claim everything back that you can. The Return is designed to let you not only declare your income on which you may be taxed, but also to set out your expenses against which you can claim money back.

The new self-assessment Income Tax Returns are long and may look very daunting. However, there are many useful leaflets you can obtain from the Inland Revenue and from the various organisations listed at the back of this book, that will help you if you find your tax situation confusing. If you are elderly, disabled or widowed, organisations like Age Concern, RADAR and CRUSE will help you with the practical details. If you are not in any of those categories, then you could go to the nearest Citizens Advice

Bureau for help or you could buy a book to guide you through all the details. *Check Your Tax*, published annually by Foulsham contains all the relevant information. However, please remember that the Inland Revenue are not ogres, they are there to help you and, providing you are not trying to evade paying tax, your local tax office personnel will gladly sit down with you and go through the details of your income and give you sound advice.

If your income is large enough to warrant it, you may, of course wish to employ an accountant to do all the hard work for you. This should cost you around £300 per year.

For the purposes of tax assessment there are various types of income, some of which are taxable and some not. When you fill in a tax return you have to declare all sources of income and the Inland Revenue will ignore them or assess tax as necessary.

Make a list of all your sources of income (see Chapter 4). They should fall into one of the following categories:

Income where tax has already been deducted

- Building society, bank and Giro deposit accounts

- Interest from shares in British companies

- Income from annuities (more about these later)

- Interest on Local Authority loans

- Interest on Government Gilt Edged Securities

Income which should also have tax deducted at source (check, particularly in the case of casual employment)

- Earnings from full-time, part-time or casual employment

🐾 Pensions from previous employments or from deceased spouse's employer

Income from which tax will not have been deducted

🐾 Industrial death benefit

🐾 Unemployment and supplementary benefits (not taxable for women who are over the age of 60)

🐾 National Insurance retirement pension (State old age pension)

🐾 Widows' pensions, widows' allowance

🐾 Business profits from self-employment or partner-ship (including things like catalogue agencies and football pools collection if they exceed your personal allowances)

🐾 Rental income from letting property

🐾 Interest from bank investment accounts

🐾 Interest on ordinary National Savings Accounts (not deposit accounts)

🐾 Income from abroad (shares, pensions, etc.)

🐾 Income from trusts

🐾 Repayments of insurance policies within the first four years of the policies' life

🐾 Interest from Government Securities purchased through the Post Office

🐾 Interest from loans you make to other people

Income that is exempt from tax

- Education grants and awards

- Winnings from betting, football pools, The National Lottery and premium bonds

- Strike pay

- Social Security Benefits (note that not all Social Security Benefits are exempt from tax and the criteria keep changing. Read more about benefits later in the chapter and check with your local tax office regarding your tax position if you claim benefits)

- Redundancy pay (up to £30,000)

- Home Improvement Grants (not loans)

- Compensation for loss of office or position awarded by a tribunal (up to £30,000)

- Interest and bonuses on National Savings Certificates and the Save As You Earn scheme

- Interest from Index-linked Savings Certificates

- Interest on delayed tax repayments

- Alimony maintenance payments received. The rules cover not only cash payments but also the settlement of household bills

- TESSA (Tax Exempt Special Savings Account). The Government introduced them to encourage saving but they are restricted to one per person aged 18 or over who can save up to £9,000 over 5 years. TESSAs can earn unusually high interest and at the end of 5 years you receive your original investment back plus all the interest, without any tax being payable, but interest rates are not guaranteed over the 5 years – they can go down!

Now take a look at your outgoings: there are some expenses which can be set against tax, such as

- Interest on certain loans. The qualifying limit for house purchase loans and for loans to persons aged 65 and over to purchase life annuities secured on their main residence is £30,000

- Charitable covenants. Covenanted donations to charities for a term of more than three years can be offset against tax if you are someone who pays the higher rate of tax

- Employees who donate up to £1200 per year to charity through their pay at work will receive tax relief on that amount under a payroll giving scheme

- Expenses against earnings. Expenses incurred as part of a job, or as a self-employed person, can be offset, providing the necessary receipts are kept and the type of expense is allowable. Check with your tax office

- Fees or subscriptions to necessary professional organisations, e.g. to the BMA if you are a doctor, can be offset

- Life assurance premiums. Tax relief is given as pre 15 March 1984 policies, 12.5 per cent of the total premium

SOCIAL SECURITY BENEFITS

The Social Security system is not a charity. Many truly deserving individuals do not realise what they are entitled to claim or are too misguidedly proud to take a benefit which is actually their right. You or your parents have paid into the system for many years, so you are entitled to claim when you are in need.

If you want more detailed information on benefits you can ring any one of the network of Social Security offices across the country. You can find the telephone number of your local office in the directory, listed under Benefits Agency or Social Security. There are many useful leaflets at your local Social Security office and sometimes in your local post office, Citizens Advice Bureau and doctor's surgery. If you are in straitened circumstances, please ask for help. You cannot know whether you are eligible for financial help unless you ask.

GRANTS FOR THOSE IN NEED

Please do not gloss over this section, because you never know when your circumstances may change and you find yourself in need – particularly when you are elderly or become ill. A friend of mine, who had worked all her life and thought she had amassed a comfortable nest-egg for her old age, became ill with crippling arthritis and she found that, over a period of ten years, all her savings were eaten up and she found life a struggle financially after that.

No matter how careful you are with money and how much you plan for the future, sometimes life can deal a cruel blow for which no one can prepare.

There are certain organisations that make grants for needy situations. These have to be applied for through a social worker at your local social services department. The grants can vary in amounts from £25 to £2,000 and cover a variety of needs, from buying essential equipment, such as telephones or medical aids, to covering the cost of convalescence after illness or a much-needed holiday for someone who is on a very low income.

There is a publication called *A Guide to Grants for Individuals in Need* which you should be able to read at your local reference library.

GRANTS FOR THE DISABLED OR ILL

There are many grant-making charities that may be able to assist financially, if you have the relevant illness or disability with which they are concerned. Again, the contact has to be made through a social worker:

ALZHEIMER'S DISEASE SOCIETY

ARTHRITIS CARE ELECTRONIC

AIDS FOR THE BLIND

ACTION FOR BLIND PEOPLE

THE ALFRED DE ROTHSCHILD CHARITY *(for people unable to pay in full for medical treatment of a special nature)*

THE MARGARET DE SOUSA DEIRO FUND *(for gentlewomen with tuberculosis or other diseases)*

INVALIDS AT HOME MOTABILITY *(provides cars and powered wheelchairs at low cost)*

THE FLORENCE NIGHTINGALE AID-IN-SICKNESS TRUST

THE ADA OLIVER WILL TRUST *(for people with cancer or rheumatism)*

THE NATIONAL TRUSS AND SURGICAL APPLIANCE SOCIETY *(for disabled people's mobility needs, independence and earning power aids, such as computers)*

THE STROKE ASSOCIATION

Grants for the Elderly

The following grant-making charities may be able to assist you financially. These also require an approach made through a social worker.

THE CARE TRUST COUNSEL AND CARE OF THE ELDERLY

FRIENDS OF THE ELDERLY AND GENTLEFOLK'S HELP

THE NATIONAL BENEVOLENT INSTITUTION

HOME WARMTH FOR THE AGED

THE ROYAL UNITED KINGDOM BENEFICENT ASSOCIATION

THE UNIVERSAL BENEFICENT SOCIETY

S C WITTING TRUST FAMILY WELFARE ASSOCIATION

THE UNITY FUND FOR THE ELDERLY

THE SAINSBURY FAMILY CHARITABLE TRUSTS

THE R L GLASSPOOL CHARITY TRUST

THE LUBRICTORS CHARITABLE TRUST

Grants for Women

Most of these charities were set up in the Victorian era when women on their own faced genuine hardship if they lost the financial protection of their family or husband. Therefore, some of the criteria seem a little quaint and may cause you to smile.

Some of the charities were set up during the First World War, when women began to have careers and there was a noticeable upsurge in the number of spinsters because a huge number of men were killed in the War. Working professional women in those days did not have pension schemes. In fact most women were not included at all in company pension schemes until it was made law in the late 1970s. Therefore, there are, now, many elderly women who are not as well-off as they could be in retirement.

Some of these organisations can be approached directly

by individuals, but may need an endorsement by a health professional.

THE FREDERICK ANDREW CONVALESCENT TRUST
Grants range from £150 to £500 and are for convalescence after an illness for professional women who are working or retired.

THE BROADLANDS HOME TRUST
Offers regular allowances of £4 a week for widows and spinsters in poor circumstances but not in residential care; small grants for books and clothes for girls for further training. One-off grants range from £50 to £100.

THE DEAKIN INSTITUTION
Ladies who live in the UK, have never been married, who are in reduced circumstances and are members of the Church of England or of a church having full membership of the Council of Churches for Britain and Ireland. Grants are not usually given to ladies under 55 years of age. These are in the form of annuities, usually £260 a year, paid half-yearly.

THE ARTHUR TOWNROW PENSIONS FUND
Spinsters in England over 40 years of age who are in need, of good character and are members of the Church of England or of a Protestant dissenting church that acknowledges the doctrine of the Holy

---

Trinity. The charity grants about 360 regular allowances of £5 a week. One half of the pensions must be paid to women living in Derbyshire but the remaining grants may be paid anywhere in England to any women over 40 years of age with an income of less than £3,865 a year.

THE MARGARET DE SOUSA DEIRO FUND
For women with tuberculosis and other diseases. The grants are for extra comforts, warm clothing, nourishment, heating, convalescence, etc. Usually between £100 and £300.

THE ANNIE ARBIB TRUST
One-off and recurrent grants for Jewish women in need. A letter of recommendation from a social worker or similar professional is required.

THE CROSSLEY FUND
These grants are for help with rent only for poor widows and spinsters of at least 50 years of age. Very small amounts of up to £2.50 a week.

THE NORTHERN LADIES ANNUITY SOCIETY
Grants for ladies over the age of 65, who live in the North of England and have an annual income of no more than £6,000. Annual grants are paid quarterly and range from £260 to £520 per year. Cold weather and Christmas grants may also be given.

THE PERRY FUND
Grants for single elderly ladies from professional families, whether widows or unmarried.

ST ANDREWS SOCIETY FOR LADIES IN NEED
Single elderly ladies (aged over 60) from a well-educated and/or professional background who are in reduced circumstances. Regular weekly grants from £5 to £10 a week; special grants towards heating costs, moving expenses, medication, etc.; holiday grants to help with convalescent holidays.

THE ROYAL SOCIETY FOR THE RELIEF OF INDIGENT GENTLEWOMEN OF SCOTLAND
Regular yearly allowances of £520 and up to £900 for needy widowed or unmarried gentlewomen over 50 years of age of Scottish birth or education who have a professional or business background. Occasional one-off grants have been given for holidays, telephones, TV licences, nursing costs, etc.

THE SOCIETY FOR THE ASSISTANCE OF LADIES IN REDUCED CIRCUMSTANCES
Grants for elderly and infirm ladies living on their own who are low incomes. Monthly allowances of up to £10 per week to assist ladies who are living in their own homes.

STUDENTS

Independent students (i.e. those who are over 25 years of age or have supported themselves for 3 years prior to enrolling for study) get the same basic rate of means-tested living accommodation grant as younger students who are living away from home.

If you are disabled you can get extra allowances if your disability makes it more expensive for you to take your course. The allowances are means-tested and are to cover the following:

- The assistance of a non-medical personal helper.

- Major items of special equipment.

- Other extra costs. This is usually to cover minor items such as tape or braille paper, or it can be used to top up the other two allowances.

Means Testing for Grants

Some of your income will affect the amount of grant you receive. But some of your income is exempt and will not affect your grant. The exact figures that apply change from year to year, so check with your local education authority first. For the purposes of means testing they will ignore:

- Some of the income from any scholarship.

- Some of your income from your permanent employers, if they release you, for example, on full- or part-time pay.

- Any income from casual or part-time jobs during your course; this includes work during the holidays, in the evening or at weekends.

- Part of any trust income, depending on your circumstances.

- Part of any pension; this does not include disability pensions.

✿ Any social security payments or other similar payments which are not taxed.

✿ Any educational payments such as student loans or payments from your college's Access Funds (more about that later).

✿ Some of your income from any other sources e.g. alimony from an ex-husband.

However, the whole amount of your income from all sources will be assessed, along with your outgoings, if you are supporting yourself.

Student Loans

These are loans, which the Government funds, to help you meet your living costs. The Student Loans Company administers the loans scheme. To qualify for a loan you must be a full-time student aged less than 50 when your course starts. You must also have a bank or building society account that can accept direct credits and pay direct debits. You must also undertake to tell the Students Loans Company if you stop attending your course before finishing it or finish earlier than you intended, because you will then have to start repaying your loan. You can only apply for a loan once in each academic year of your course and for only one course at a time.

Access Funds

Colleges receive Access Funds so that they can provide selective help to certain students who have serious financial difficulties or whose access to higher education might be inhibited because of financial reasons. The size of the Funds is limited.

Career Development Loans

If you are over the age of 18 and you cannot get a full mandatory award or any other funding to help pay for the course you want to do, you may be able to apply for a Career Development Loan. The Employment Department manages CDLs through a partnership with a number of High Street banks. They can support courses in a wide range of vocational areas.

A CDL is designed to cover course fees and other costs such as books, materials, childcare and, if the course is full-time, living expenses.

Sponsorship

One final source of income for students is the possibility of a scholarship or bursary. There is a book called *Sponsorship for Students* which is published by the Careers and Occupational Information Centre (COIC). It lists all scholarships and bursaries that awarded by charities, colleges, trusts and businesses and gives advice on how to qualify for such awards and how to apply. You should be able to find the book in any good reference library.

Having investigated all possible sources of income, you are now ready to turn your attention to managing your money.

Managing Your Money

*I*t's no good checking every last drop of your income, of course, if it isn't enough to cover your expenditure. If you are to feel comfortable, you must be sure that what comes in at least equals what's going out. To be certain of this, you will have to make a few lists and do a few sums. Like everything else I have suggested, it's not difficult, and although it may take you some time, it will be worth it for peace of mind.

BALANCING YOUR BOOKS

Take a large sheet of paper and write on the top left-hand side '**Income**'. Underneath this heading, list anything which brings you in an income. Such as:

> Salary (full-time)
> Salary (part-time)
> Interest on savings
> Interest on shares
> Company bonus (if it's a regular guaranteed one)
> Commission
> Rents from lodgers/holiday lets

Other rent (say, on a garage you rent out)
Tips
Royalties
Profit-sharing scheme
Alimony/maintenance payments
Student grant
Allowance from parents
Holiday job
Trust income
Annuity payments
State benefits
State retirement pension
Private employment pension
Disability pension from work
Services pension (Army etc.)
Repayments on loans you have made to others

At the top of the right-hand side of the page write the heading '**Expenses**' and list underneath that heading all of your outgoings. Your list will probably look something like this, although not all the items will be applicable to you:

Mortgage
Rent
Council tax
Ground rent
Service charges
Gas
Electricity
Other heating expenses (paraffin, bottled gas, etc.)
Telephone
Water rates
Communal heating charges (if in rented accomodation)

House contents insurance
Health insurance
Life insurance
Mortgage indemnity insurance
Electrical appliance insurance
Building insurance
Pet insurance (for vets' fees)
Car insurance
Car tax
Car maintenance
Car MOT
Pension plan
Investments
Food (including toiletries and cleaning items)
Drink (alcohol etc.)
TV rental
TV licence
Video rental
Meals out (from staff canteen to evenings out)
Fares to and from work and college
Club fees
Loan repayments
Domestic help wages
Care package
Mobility payments
Savings

Now calculate your income amounts and expense amounts in monthly sums. For example, if you pay approximately £50 a quarter for your telephone bill, then round it up to £60 (it helps if you overestimate the expenditure) and break it down to the monthly sum of £20. If you are paid a weekly wage, then add it up to the monthly total and put that down, and so on. Then write the relevant sums by the relevant items as in Figure 1.

FIGURE 1 INCOME VERSUS EXPENDITURE
FOR MRS A, A WIDOW AGED 47

Income per month		Expenditure per month	
Salary (before tax)	380.00	Council tax	18
Savings interest (taxed)	5.00	Water rates	7
Tips	30.00	Gas	20
Catalogue commission	25.00	Electricity	20
Widows pension	164.60	Fares	20
(before tax)		Building insurance	8
		Contents insurance	6
		Food	100
		Drink	30
		TV rental	20
		Telephone	15
		Savings	50
		Health insurance	50
		Golf club fee	10
		HP repayments	30
Gross income	604.60	Total	404
Net income	509.16*		

*Mrs A. is allowed to earn approximately £217.83 per month without paying tax, leaving a balance of £381.77 each month that is liable for 25% tax deduction. That means that approximately £95.44 would be deducted, leaving the net income each month of £509.16.

As you can see from Figure 1, Mrs A has a healthy surplus income of £105.16 each month.

Draw up a plan of your spending throughout the year, which will show the periods when you are likely to have a lot of bills coming in. You will then be able to see how long you are likely to have in between to put money aside for the tough months. It should look like Figure 2.

FIGURE 2 CASHFLOW FOR 199_

	Jan	Feb	Mar	Apr	May	Jun	Jul	Aug	Sep	Oct	Nov	Dec
Mortgage/Rent	*	*	*	*	*	*	*	*	*	*	*	*
Council Tax	*			*	*	*	*	*	*	*	*	*
Water Rates				*					*			
Gas		*			*			*			*	
Electricity		*			*			*			*	
Telephone	*			*			*			*		
HP Repayments	*	*	*	*	*	*	*	*	*	*	*	*
TV/Video Rental	*	*	*	*	*	*	*	*	*	*	*	*
House Insurances – Buildings			*									
Contents								*				
Other Insurances – Health Scheme	*											
Life					*							
Car Expenses – Tax								*				
Insurance				*								
Service										*		
MOT										*		
Miscellaneous												
Totals												

Fill in the chart with the actual amounts you spend. You may of course have to put in some estimates in the first year. Use the miscellaneous sections to fill in the cost of holidays, Christmas, etc. and also unexpected large bills, such as car repairs.

Make a new chart every year, filling in the date at the top. Keep all the charts safely.

As you fill in the amounts, your cashflow charts will give you a historical record of what you actually spend. You can then use this to identify months of heavy expenditure so that you can be prepared. You can also use it to forecast future spending. You will know what certain amounts will be, but others will have to be estimated, by adding, say, 10 per cent, on to last year's bill.

Of course, your budget and your yearly cashflow projection may be totally different from the above examples. You may not be a salaried person at all, you may be a retired person with no mortgage left to pay. Whatever your circumstances, the point is that you should have enough money coming in in the 'Income' column to meet the outgoings in the 'Expenses' column with, hopefully, a bit left over for rainy days and holidays. By breaking down the quarterly or annual outgoings into monthly amounts, you will see exactly how much money you have to set aside every month to meet those periodic demands on your cash.

STAYING WITHIN YOUR INCOME – OR BOOSTING IT

If your income does not exceed your expenditure, then you must isolate items on your expenditure list first of all, to see if they can be reduced. For example, the food bill – are you spending unwisely? Be realistic about your needs. Do not skimp on food and heating or you may put your life at risk in the winter, particularly if you are elderly or disabled. On the other hand, if you are in the habit of buying Marks & Spencer's ready-made meals, packets of smoked salmon, hand-made chocolates or anything else that takes your fancy, then this is an area where you could indulge yourself less and make some sensible economies.

Be practical about your situation. If you are sitting on your own in a very large house, which is draining away your resources because it still has mortgage payments to be met and it takes a lot of money to heat and light every year, you must seriously consider cashing in your assets by moving to a smaller house that eliminates your mortgage and cuts down on running costs, or by taking out an annuity on your house.

An annuity, as explained in an earlier chapter, (see page 44) is an arrangement with a financial institution whereby, if you are over retirement age and do not want to leave your property to anyone when you die, they will effectively buy your house from you (albeit at less than the market value), give you guaranteed security of tenure until you die, and turn the money that they pay you for the house into a regular income for the rest of your life. These schemes have rejuvenated many elderly people's lives and effectively eliminated their money worries.

If you are younger, perhaps living alone after the death of an elderly parent, or are widowed, and you are in the same situation of having a large house or flat that is too much of a financial burden for you, then you could sell, or consider taking in paying guests. Better to do either of those things than spend the next few years in a state of anxiety and misery because of money worries. As other chapters in this book show, you can make a marvellous home for yourself somewhere else, providing you choose with care.

If you are renting accommodation and suspect that the rent is too high, you can apply to a rent tribunal to have it reduced. The council tax can be queried and even contested through a tribunal although, in practice, few people are successful in getting it reduced. The tax is based on a valuation of the property, and this can be challenged through the local Valuation Office. As a person living alone you should be entitled to a Single Person Discount of 25 per cent, but this is not granted automatically, so make sure you apply for it. If you are on a low income, you may also be able to get help with paying your Council Tax by applying for Council Tax Benefit, which is means-tested.

If you are working, then why not look for a job that pays more or a job that pays the same but reduces your travelling costs? Or ask your employer if you can change your hours of work so that you can take advantage of cheap rate travel? Merely by working from ten until six, instead of nine to five, workers living ten miles from London can save half their travel costs per week.

Or, if you are young and fit enough, you could take a second job at weekends, or some evenings. Perhaps just for a while, to tide you over a particularly bad crop of bills. Evening work can be found in fast-food chains, cinemas, theatres, pubs, discos, restaurants, garages, and supermarkets. If you have a skill – typing, or knowledge of motor mechanics for instance – try advertising locally for weekend work. Simple things like window-cleaning or car-washing can be quite lucrative. Do you have a hobby that you can cash in on? Craft work, such as hand knitting or celebration cake decorating, can sell quite well.

BEING THRIFTY

Some of the ways in which you can be thrifty with food will be covered in Chapter 6 and home energy management, discussed in Chapter 5 should make a significant difference to your heating bills this winter.

There are many other ways of being thrifty. For example, although in Chapter 5, I advocate a policy of not hoarding rubbish, there is a difference when it comes to saving useful items that help towards thrift. If you save plastic containers that come into the house – margarine tubs, yoghurt pots – you will not need to buy plastic containers for the freezer, or proper flowerpots. I even save certain tins! I have a tin-opener that cuts off the whole top of the tin under the rim and leaves a blunt edge. I then wash the tins, paint and decorate the outsides and use them as cache pots for all my plants, which neatly disguises the yoghurt pots in which I have planted them!

You can also save paper and plastic bags and use them again and again for lunch sandwiches. (Making and taking your own lunches to work is a very big saving in itself.)

There are also more important economies. The telephone bill. Ask for a tariff of telephone charges from your telephone company. This will show you how much you can save on your bill if you make calls out of peak periods. You can buy a telephone logging device (they start at around £30) which will tell you how long each telephone call you make is and how much it costs. It will enable you to challenge telephone bills if you think they are wrong and to gain a better idea of how much you are paying while you talk. However, if you have a touch-tone phone, you can obtain call charge information quite simply by using certain keys on your phone. You can use this service for all calls or just a single call now and then. Full details of this service can be found in your telephone directory which also provides pricing information and details of all BT services and customer helpline numbers.

Nowadays there is hot competition between the phone service suppliers, who all offer different discount schemes. The best known of these offers a reduction on your five most frequently dialled numbers. They also all have different rates for long distance and international calls, so it is well worth shopping around to find out who has the best deals for you. Do bear in mind, though, that if you use a supplier other than BT, you will have to pay for the use of the line and you may have to buy a new phone if yours is not equipped to offer all these new services

Do not stop using the telephone altogether just to save money, it is important that you maintain social contacts, but how about occasionally writing a letter instead? You can say as much as you like in a letter and it will not cost you any more than the price of a stamp.

Look hard at your outgoings and see if you can eliminate any luxuries without making yourself too miserable. Will you be unhappy without a video? Would it be more sensible in the long run to buy a second-hand television rather than to keep renting one? How many clubs do you belong to that you never really visit? How many magazines do you subscribe to at which you hardly ever glance? Do you really need a newspaper every day? Perhaps you could read a library book on the train instead – library books cost nothing unless they are overdue. If you have your hair done once a week, could you set it yourself and just visit the hairdresser's for a cut every two months? If you smoke, could you try very hard to give it up and save all that money? Do you feed your pet unnecessarily expensive food and could you buy a cheaper alternative? If you like plants and gardening, could you try propagating your own from cuttings rather than buying more? Or could you ask about taking cuttings or divisions from neighbours' plants?

Having flowers in the house is lovely, but fresh flowers can be rather expensive; artificial arrangements would save money in the long run and still give you a splash of colour. Could you grow your own vegetables and fruit? This represents an enormous saving and the taste is better than shop-bought.

Earn interest on your money whenever possible. Do not keep money at home in tins or piggy banks, start savings accounts with the post office, banks or building societies. Instead of buying television licence stamps every month, put the same amount of money into a savings account, then you will at least earn some interest on it throughout the year. But make sure it is the kind of account that allows you to get your money out when you need it.

Look at your banking arrangements. The banks are becoming more competitive and you should shop around to get the best deal, especially if you are being charged for the administration of standing orders and direct debits, or you have a loan or overdraft facility.

As I mentioned earlier in this chapter, check that you are paying the right amount of tax and, now that we all have to use the IR self-assessment scheme, make sure that you fill in your tax forms correctly and on time, otherwise you could end up paying unnecessary tax or interest. Don't pay for expensive financial advice, unless you run your own business or have large investments to manage. Any Inland Revenue office will help you, free of charge, to make sense of your tax forms and fill them in correctly.

Little economies, when they are added up, come to quite a lot of money each month. The above are a few ideas; really only you can be the best judge of where and how you can be more thrifty.

CONTROLLING YOUR MONEY

Beware of over-enthusiastic financial organisations. The only way to keep control of money is to handle it yourself. I always prefer to pay all my bills by cheque or by cash. I hate direct debits and standing orders – but that is just me. For many people, standing orders and direct debits are a good way of having control over their outgoings. However, whatever your preferred banking arrangements are, let me urge you to check your bank statements in minute detail. Banks are not infallible and they can certainly make expensive mistakes sometimes.

The method, favoured by so many elderly people, of keeping little tins in the house marked 'rent', 'telephone', 'gas', etc. into which you put money each week, may give you a certain amount of satisfaction as a way of saving, but, apart from the fact that, as I mentioned earlier, your money is not making interest if you keep it at home, it will also be a nice little present for a burglar to have everything so conveniently marked and to hand for him. Never stash money in the house – whether it be in little tins, jars or under the mattress – except for a small amount for use in emergencies. If you want to divide your money into separate bill categories, have a post office book for each category. Take all your books and pay the necessary amounts into them, at intervals. It may not make you very popular with the queue behind you in the post office, but if it helps you, it does not matter.

INSURANCE AND ASSURANCE

It is completely untrue to say that there is no such thing as being over-insured, this is nonsense. Insurance is only valuable if it serves a purpose. For example, the retired single person with no surviving family has absolutely no need of anything other than a minimal life assurance to cover funeral expenses etc. (Sorry to sound morbid.) For such a person, health insurance is valuable but an expensive life assurance is not.

The difference between assurance and insurance is that the former is a guarantee to pay money on the death of the named person or, in some cases, earlier during the person's lifetime, and the latter is an undertaking by an insurance company to undertake the risks of repaying cash for any loss or damage, in return for regular premiums.

There are many different kinds of insurance and assurance. I have set out below short notes on the commonest types. Be sure you understand what each is for and whether it is necessary in your individual circumstances before you decide to take out any policy.

Home Insurances

Building insurance: Most lenders of money, e.g. banks and building societies, insist that a house owner takes out an insurance for the worth of the building, to protect against it being accidentally destroyed. The insurance should cover fixed outbuildings but, as many people found out during the hurricane of 1987, it does not cover fences.

Mortgage indemnity insurance: This is an insurance that repays the mortgage in full should the person paying the mortgage die.

House contents insurance: This insures your furniture, carpets, clothes, in fact anything authorised to be in the house, against damage or theft. 'Authorised' is the important word because there is a famous case of an insurance company turning down a claim for a new kitchen damaged by fire when they discovered that a motorbike was in the kitchen at the time, being stripped down.

Maisonette indemnity insurance: This is required for owners of flats and maisonettes. In simple terms, the insurance protects the value of your home against any action or inaction, by another owner in your shared building, that may devalue your property. If, for example, your downstairs neighbour allows his flat to become damp and infested with woodworm so that it affects your property, then you can claim against the insurance.

Valuables insurance: If you keep valuables in the home, such as jewellery or antiques, you need a special insurance and a professional valuation of the objects. Valuables can be added to the house contents insurance.

Mortgage protection insurance: This is a recent introduction which covers mortgage payments in the case of redundancy, usually for a specified period of time.

Life Assurance

This is broken up into three basic types:

Term assurance: This covers a person's life for a specified term – usually to cover the cost of something should you die prematurely, e.g. the mortgage, if you should die before it is repaid, or your function in a company if you are very important (sometimes called Keyman insurance). It is not a form of saving, as you lose the premium money if you survive the term.

Endowment assurance: This is a form of saving as your life will be covered for a fixed term and, at the end of it, you will be paid a fixed amount, plus bonuses. Many people use this form of assurance as a method of financing a house purchase. In other words, a building society will accept the policy as a guarantee of repayment of the capital sum at the end of the term, and in the meantime you pay interest each month to the building society.

Whole life assurance: This policy does not have a fixed term, but lasts throughout the whole of a person's life, paying out to beneficiaries after his or her death.

Car Insurance

Car insureance is compulsory by law, but the legal minimum required is only that you have a 'third party' policy which covers the cost of repairs to the other person's car or property if you have an accident. However, you have the option of taking out additional forms of cover if you wish.

Third Party, Fire and Theft: This covers damage to a driver and car that is inflicted by you, and damage to your car in the case of fire or theft only. It does not cover your car for damage in an accident, and therefore it is usually the sort of insurance taken out by people whose car is worth very little.

Comprehensive: Everything is covered under this policy, including all claims for damage, fire or theft. It is the most expensive policy, but it should guarantee your peace of mind. If you car is fairly new, this is the kind of cover you should consider.

Extras – these require additional premiums:

- Windscreen cover (the cost of a replacement windscreen is covered).

- Extra driver (if you want to nominate someone who can drive your car in your place, such as a friend or relative).

- Legal costs (this covers the costs of legal representation in the case of an accident etc.).

- Replacement car – usually taken out by people whose car is a vital part of their job. It provides the cost of a replacement car if yours is off the road for any reason.

Breakdown insurance: This is what you take out when you join the AA or RAC. Your annual membership fee covers you for various grades of breakdown services (a must for women on their own). There is the basic service for when you break down away from home, or you can have the more expensive 'home start' service for the times when your car decides it will not move from your home.

Motorbike insurance: This is compulsory but pedal cycle insurance is not, although there are policies available. If you use a bicycle a lot, you should make sure that it is insured as they are so easy to steal. You can do this as part of you house contents insurance.

Motor insurance policy premiums should reduce over several years if you accrue 'No claims bonuses', in other words, if you do not make any claims for damage, etc. Many insurance companies now are offering cheaper deals to older drivers, as statistics have proved that younger drivers are responsible for most of the accidents in the UK. Shop around and get the best deal you can or get an insurance broker to do this for you. It can vary by as much as £100 from one insurance company to another.

Health Insurance

This comes in many packages, so, as with all insurance, shop around. You can cover yourself for certain kinds of private medical treatment, including hospital stays, and you can cover yourself so that you would receive an income if you should fall sick and be unable to work.

In some policies you can elect to do both, and in others you only receive cash if you take NHS treatment instead of private. There are exceptions. Health insurance companies will not cover alcohol- or drug-related illnesses, AIDS-related illnesses or psychiatric care. Neither will they cover what is called a 'pre-condition', i.e. some illness or condition that existed before you took out the policy. Maternity or dentistry is not usually covered, although some separate policies are surfacing now which specifically cover such things. There is often an upper age limit for policyholders, although, in recent years, the insurance companies have extended these upwards a little. Usually they will not accept anyone over the age of 70. Anyway, the premiums become progressively more expensive as you grow older.

Pet health insurance: This works in the same way as human health insurance. You pay the premiums and the insurance company pays the vets' bills. Usually, you have to pay the first £10 of any bill, or whatever the company nominates. And some of the companies do not pay for drugs or routine vaccinations.

Again, as with humans, 'pre-conditions' in pets are not covered. You can also elect to cover the life, theft or loss of the animal and the cost of its replacement, if it is a pedigree dog or cat or a valuable horse.

An additional – and I think, very necessary – part of most pet insurance policies is cover against the cost of damages should your animal cause an accident, for example by running out into the road

Accident insurance: This usually covers death, loss of limbs, eyes or permanent disablement, temporary disablement and expenses for hospital stays. Most people only ever take out such an insurance when they travel abroad by aeroplane.

Others

Appliance insurance: Cookers, washing machines, storage heaters, microwaves, dishwashers, tumble driers, refrigerators, freezers (including contents), music centres, videos, cleaners, televisions, computers, in other words any kind of domestic appliance is eligible for appliance insurance.

Personal money and credit cards: It is possible to cover yourself up to a specified limit for the loss or theft or fraudulent use of money and credit cards. Cover is usually for the United Kingdom and abroad. Travellers cheques are automatically insured, of course. Some credit cards also automatically insure goods recently bought with the credit card against loss, theft or damage within a specified period of the purchase.

Travel insurance: This should cover theft or loss of baggage, medical expenses abroad, loss or theft of valuables/money/travellers cheques and unavoidable cancellation of your holiday.

The list above covers the main insurance categories. There are various packages with various names. It really is important to decide whether you really need certain insurances or whether you can do without them. Then examine all the available packages and read the fine print.

For example, with health insurance, you must compare all of the packages on offer to get the best deal, because the benefits can be markedly different.

In the end, it is possible, technically, to insure against any risk. You can make a private deal with insurance companies to insure your legs for a million pounds if they are essential to how you earn your living!

BANKING ARRANGEMENTS

When you live alone, quick and convenient access to your

money is exceptionally important, because you do not have a live-in partner, flatmate or family to borrow from if the need suddenly arises. Borrowing money from colleagues at work, from the petty cash box or from neighbours is a fast way of making yourself unpopular. So, make sure that you have enough money at all times – after all, it is just a question of organisation.

Although I have stressed that one should not keep large amounts of money at home, it is of value to have at least a small amount of emergency money carefully hidden somewhere in the house, say, £50. If you are housebound for any reason, perhaps snowed in, or in bed with flu, you need to be able to pay for certain items, like prescription charges which neighbours may fetch for you.

Ease of access to money has been transformed in the last few years. Not only are there cash machines at most banks and building societies, there are now cash machines at large supermarkets and shopping centres. Most cash machines are networked so that they dispense money for more than one organisation.

In addition, if you have a Switch card, or a credit card which is linked in to your bank account, such as Mastercard or Visa, all the major supermarkets now operate a 'cash-back' system, which means that when you pay for your shopping you can also ask for a certain amount of cash which will be debited immediately from your account. This is not a loan of money, for which you pay interest, it is simply another way of extracting your own money from your bank account. A Switch card can be used to pay for goods and the cost of those goods are debited immediately from your account. Retailers prefer Switch rather than cheques because they get their money immediately via computer transfer and do not have to wait for a cheque to clear.

It is possible, with a credit card, to borrow money from the credit card company through a cash machine. This is money that you do not have. It will be added to your credit card debt and you will be charged interest on it if you do not pay it back within a certain period. Some credit cards charge interest immediately on cash withdrawn in this way. Make sure you know which system applies to your credit card.

Throughout this book, I have extolled the virtues of the post office, mainly because even in the most rural areas you are likely to have a sub-post office, where you will be able to deposit and withdraw money all week and on Saturday mornings as well. The Post Office, of course, operates its own cheque account scheme – Giro – which means that you can have full banking facilities.

Where you have your main account depends very much on where you are most of the time. If, for example, you work in a town and live outside a town, it makes sense to have your account near your place of work, so that you can sort out any problems, or have interviews with your bank manager, during your lunch hour. If you had your bank near your home then it would mean taking time off work to deal with money problems. Nowadays, however, it is possible to do a lot of your banking business over the telephone and many banks offer a 24-hour telephone banking service.

Where you keep the major portion of your money depends upon what additional services you are likely to require. If you feel that, over the years, you may wish to avail yourself of some loans for home improvement, a new car, or other major item of expenditure, then you really do need to keep favour with a bank. If you have a lot of standing orders or direct debits, banks still have more experience in administering these, although building societies are catching up.

You may want a permanent overdraft facility. This is extremely useful if you are self-employed and your income fluctuates. All banks now offer 'budget accounts', which are a form of savings and overdraft system, whereby you undertake to allow the bank to transfer a set sum from your main account into your budget account each month. This accumulates and is used to pay bills. If there is any excess money in the account, it earns interest. If it goes into the red, you pay some interest. For some people it is a useful way of letting the bank take the strain of dealing with bills; others prefer to handle their own budget.

Bank and building society managers are supposed to be approachable; if yours is not, then change to another branch. As a woman on your own you need a sympathetic ear when talking over money matters. Do not allow yourself to be patronised or dismissed without proper attention.

DEALING WITH DEBT

Hopefully, you will never be in this situation if you have made a realistic appraisal of your incomings and outgoings and taken measures to raise the former and reduce the latter. Always check your bank balance, and keep a chart, as recommended earlier in this chapter, which shows you when your heaviest bills are going to come in throughout the year. That way you can make economies or generate extra income to cover the bad months and avoid debt.

Always try and put a little bit by in a savings account, if you can, to cover yourself if you get a run of unplanned expenses.

It can be very easy to find yourself in a financial crisis through no fault of your own. Bad luck could take over. For example, you might suffer a car accident and find that the other person is not insured – it will be of little consolation to you that the offender is prosecuted, you will still be faced with unexpected bills. Or, your partner may have died and left you with debts that you were unaware of.

If you find yourself in debt, do not panic. All problems have a solution. You may need a little help and advice to find that solution but take heart and keep calm.

The main things is to communicate with your creditors. Never evade their letters or phone calls, it will only make them less amenable to your predicament. It is also important for you to discuss your problem with someone. Keeping quiet and worrying about it will only make you feel worse.

There are many people to whom you can turn for help and advice. The Citizens Advice Bureaux are used to helping people sort out their debt problems. If you are elderly or disabled and have regular contact with your social services department, they may be able to help you with loans or support. Often these people will write letters for you to your creditors, to add that little bit of official weight. CRUSE is used to helping widows with debt problems as many women find unexpected debts and other financial problems cropping up after their partner's death.

If you are working, you may be able to obtain help from

your employer or personnel officer, such as an advance on salary to get you over a debt problem, particularly if it has arisen through unforeseen circumstances and not through your own negligence.

It may distress you deeply, especially if you have never been in debt before, but do not succumb to pointless worrying. Take remedial action:

- Add up all your debts to determine the total figure.

- Work out how much money you have to spare each month.

- Divide the total figure of the debts by the amount of your spare cash each month, e.g. Total debt £350: total spare cash each month £25. Divide 350 by 25 = 14. Therefore you would be able to pay off the debt over 14 months.

- If the debt is owed to one organisation, then you must write to them, explain your problem and offer to pay off the debt in 14 instalments.

- If you owe money to several organisations, then you must calculate what you can afford to pay each organisation out of your £25 spare each month:

> The gas company £10 per month for 14 months

> The electricity company £10 per month for 14 months

> The telephone company £5 per month for 14 months.

Most organisations owed money would rather make

such an arrangement and get their money back eventually, than say goodbye to the money altogether.

Certainly, the gas companies, electricity companies, local authorities and water companies are sympathetic towards people who wish to clear their debts in this way. They all have people who deal specifically with debt problems and will be happy to sit down and talk to you.

Building societies and banks who have lent you money for your mortgage will, generally, be sympathetic if you ask to suspend your mortgage payments for a fixed period because you have been made redundant or have a crisis. They can simply add the period of lapsed payments on to the end of your mortgage term. But you must inform them in writing of the situation. Do not just avoid paying bills in the hope that you will eventually find the money. If you are seriously ill or made redundant, some mortgage protection policies will give you a breathing space.

It is the small local businesses, such as your builders, coal merchant or newsagent, who are most likely to balk at a long-term clearance of debt. Again you have another alternative: go to your bank manager and explain the problem and ask for a loan so that you can pay these people off straight away. You can then pay the bank £25 a month, except that because you will then pay interest it will probably take you 20 months to pay off the loan instead of 14.

There is also the option, if you have a credit card, to pay your debts with the credit card and then pay the credit card company back in instalments. The Consumer Association published a *Which?* report showing that long term loans from credit card companies often worked out cheaper than many bank loans. You can raise cash on a credit card too, if your local small businesses who are owed money are not geared up to be paid by credit card.

If a very close relative offers to lend you money in return for an interest-free repayment of the loan, take up the offer if you know that he or she genuinely will not miss the money. However, do not be tempted to borrow from friends or neighbours, no matter how desperate you are. Many friendships have soured because the lender loses patience with the protracted period of repayment and starts becoming difficult to deal with. And never borrow money from moneylenders, or specialist finance or credit companies as they are usually called. They charge interest way above the odds and you will be paying off the debt for several years rather than 14 months.

GETTING ADVICE

Throughout this chapter, I have emphasized the importance of putting yourself in control of your financial affairs. It is imperative that you know everything about your personal money matters and direct them yourself as far as possible so that you feel confident that you are getting the best out of your income and savings.

However, there will almost certainly be times when you feel that you do not have either the knowledge, or possibly the energy, to handle matters yourself. That is the time to ask for professional help and advice.

Advice on straightforward matters such as savings, mortgages, insurance and so on can be obtained free on any High Street. Banks and building societies all have specially trained representatives who will be pleased to explain everything about the services they offer, for example the differences between types of savings accounts or mortgage repayment schemes, without any obligation on your part. They can also provide you with masses of information leaflets which you can study in your own time before making any decision.

Similarly, insurance brokers will help you choose the policy best suited to you by phoning round and obtaining quotations on your behalf. They provide the information and expertise, they save you time and you only pay for the policy you select.

If, however, you have more complicated financial affairs – say, a large amount of money to invest or existing investments which you do not really understand – you may need to consult a financial adviser. You will have to pay for this service, either by an annual fee for agreed services, or by an hourly rate. Most will offer a free introductory session of half an hour which will give you time to explain what your needs are and to find out how much you will be charged for the service, if you decide to engage them – which you are not obliged to do.

There are two types of financial adviser: independents, who are just that, and companies who want you to invest only in their own company schemes. there is nothing sinister in this: it is rather like the difference between booking a holiday direct with a tour operator or going through a travel agent who will offer you a selection of holiday companies to choose from. Look in the Yellow Pages under Financial Advisers or get a recommendation from a friend if your prefer. Whichever you select, you must make sure that they are a member of one of the authorising bodies that oversee standards or conduct in the financial industry, e.g. the PIA or FIMBRA.

Apart from investment advice, you may think you need an accountant. Do not employ one simply because you are daunted by the prospect of completing the new 60-page self-assessment forms for the Inland Revenue. As I have already said, you can get help direct from your local tax office – their officers are very approachable, contrary to popular belief! If you really do need an accountant, check again that he or she is properly qualified and preferably use one who is recommended by someone you trust. You can, if you wish, arrange this as part of a package with your investment advisers.

Finally, as ever, the Citizens Advice Bureau can help you with advice and names and addresses of accredited financial organisations.

Your Home is Your Castle

Whether you have just moved into a new home or have been living in the same place for years, the main thing is that you are alone and you must make your home the sort of place which pleases you. For some, home is the centre of their life, their pride, their joy and their sanctuary. For others it may merely be the base from which they conduct a busy working and social life. For all of us, however, it is probably our greatest asset and deserves to be taken care of. The aim of this chapter is to provide help in making your home a comfortable, economical and secure place – and beautiful too, if you wish – for you to enjoy with friends or alone.

MAKING YOURSELF COMFORTABLE

Comfort, to me, means warmth, and whenever I move to a new home the first thing I do is to make it as warm as possible. This often means great economy too, for eliminating draughts and adding insulation will save pounds on energy bills.

The Energy Efficiency Office publish excellent advice

about making your home energy-efficient and most of the literature is available through your local council offices and electricity showrooms. Local authorities can give advice on grants that may be available.

Windows

If you are on a really stringent budget, there are many very cheap ways of making your windows less energy-draining in the winter.

Firstly, plug all the draughts with strips of foam draught excluder (quite cheap from DIY stores) but make sure that you can open and close the windows properly. You can then make your own form of secondary double glazing by buying some heavy duty clear plastic sheeting and stretching this across the inside of the window frame. You must still be able to open the window, of course, so attach it to the window surround with double-sided tape, which can be easily ripped away in an emergency, or frequently replaced if you want to open the windows to air the room. If you have multi-paned windows, you can stretch cling film across each pane. But stretch it very tight like a drum, or it will not have the effect of keeping out the cold air. Hang heavy curtains at all the windows to cut out draughts and keep in warmth, or add thermal linings to existing curtains. Have any cracked window glass replaced before the winter sets in.

If you do not have double glazing, then think about putting it in, at least for some of your windows. Secondary double glazing is quite reasonable in price and is fairly easily fitted. Armed with a saw and a screwdriver, I have fitted my own secondary units and now some companies are producing panes that are made of high resilience plastics, which are much lighter to handle and much warmer to touch than glass. Secondary double glazing involves the fitting of a wooden or plastic frame a few centimetres inside your existing window and slotting in sliding panes of glass or substitute glass. Large DIY centres stock the complete kits, which will fit any standard-sized window.

Of course, if you can afford full double-glazed replacement windows, then you have no problems, and it does actually add value to your property, providing it is in a style sympathetic to the house itself. However, it is a very expensive exercise and it will take time to recoup the expenditure, so it should not be entered into unless you are really sure that you can afford it. A word of warning about installing replacement windows – make sure that your local authority will allow you to do so. If you live in a very old property which may be listed (you would be suprised what they consider to be worth listing) or you live in a conservation area, you may not be allowed to install any replacement windows that use modern materials such as uPVC. Check first.

Doors

It is relatively easy to fit metal or plastic strips along the bottom of doors to exclude draughts and foam strips all round the door frames. The metal strips with the thick brush on the bottom are best for doors that open on to carpeted floors. Treat any panes of glass in front doors like windows and give them some form of double glazing as described above.

The external doors, of course, admit the greatest number of draughts, so apart from fitting excluders, it is also worth hanging a heavy curtain over the inside of the front and back doors. The curtain must be capable of being drawn across and back – no matter how bad the winter, you will be answering the door occasionally! Do not forget letter boxes: they can be fitted with brush-type draught excluders too, or you can fit a box on the back to catch the mail.

Radiators

Radiators are rarely used to their greatest effect. Shelves over the top of radiators push warm air down into a room, rather than letting it float immediately up to the ceiling. Fixing aluminium foil behind radiators, dull side against the wall, helps to reflect heat outwards, instead of letting it be absorbed by the wall. If you are moving into a new home and you have a bit of spare cash, you may like to consider having certain radiators repositioned. Often, they are placed directly under windows and at least 30 per cent of the heat is wasted by just going out through the window glass. Think about this carefully though and take advice, as there may be restrictions on where you can place the radiator and it will use up wall space.

Lofts

When all the draughts that bring cold air in are blocked off, you then need to insulate in order to keep warmth in. As much as 25 per cent of home heat is lost through an uninsulated roof. In most cases, providing the timbers in your roof are sound and you can walk about up there, it is not a difficult job to insulate a loft. You can do it yourself or get a price from a local home maintenance firm.

There are two types of loft insulation you can buy in

large DIY stores – insulating mats, which are thermal wadding which comes in large rolls, and loose granular material, which comes in sacks. The mats are unrolled and laid between the joists, while the granular material is just poured on to the boards. Loft insulation should be at least 100mm (4 in) thick in order to be effective. So, if you are insulating with granules, take a ruler up there with you so that you can measure the depth as you go along. Follow all instructions on packaging as insulating material can be toxic.

All the insulation in the world won't help, of course, if your roof leaks and lets in cold air through damaged or missing roof tiles. These must be replaced first. There is also an insulating method, which can only be done by professionals, which involves spraying the whole loft with a liquid bonding material, which sets and protects against damp and heat loss at the same time.

If you have a house or a top floor flat with an uninsulated flat roof, it can be an expensive operation to insulate, as the roofing material needs to be stripped off and several layers of insulation put underneath before re-felting. Putting a layer of polystyrene, either in tile or roll form, on to the ceiling of a room under a flat roof can help, but don't do it in a kitchen. Polystyrene is extremely hazardous in cases of fire.

It is still possible to get grants from local authorities for loft insulation for certain old properties or if you are a senior citizen or disabled. Make enquiries.

Never, never part with money to so-called 'loft insulation specialists', or anyone else for that matter, who calls at the door. In many cases they are con men and many elderly ladies living alone have lost large sums of money this way. If you need advice or professional services, ask someone you trust for a recommendation.

Water Tanks and Pipes

Insulating water tanks is the next job and this can be done with special padded material, secured in place by wire, or with special ready-made padded tank jackets or, if you have a standard-sized water tank, with special pre-cut packs of sheet insulation that are placed around the tank and secured with tape or wire.

Water pipes in the loft and in any unheated room, such as a utility room, should be lagged with strips of insulating material wrapped around and around, or with special pre-formed foam insulation that fits neatly around the pipe. Tank jacket kits and pipe lagging materials are readily available at any DIY shop and fitting them yourself is quite a simple task.

Immersion heaters that are not performing efficiently can use up a great deal of energy trying to heat water. One of the biggest problems in a hard water area is limescale forming inside the heater which can make the heating element work overtime just to heat up a small amount of water. If you suspect this is happening in your cylinder, you will need the advice of a plumber.

Floors

It is estimated that 15 per cent of home heat is lost through timber floors. You may live in a modern home where the style of bare floorboards is acceptable, but nothing beats good carpeting as insulation. In an old house it may be that gaps in the skirting boards are the chief cause of heat loss and/or draughts, in which case a quick brandishing of wood filler around your home will solve the problem. You can, if you like, take up the floorboards and fill underneath with the same granular insulation material recommended for lofts, but it is a difficult job and one strictly for professionals.

Walls

The only thing left if your house or flat is still not as warm as you would like, is wall insulation. Cavity walls can be filled by a contractor who will advise you on the best type of material for your property. There has been some bad press in recent years about the use of foam in cavity wall insulation and its possible side-effects on people's health. Make sure you talk to several reputable contractors before making the final decision. Also consider the outlay in relation to the savings.

Solid walls can only really be insulated by applying a material to the exterior of the walls (rendering, cladding, pebbledash, etc.) to make the walls thicker, or by panelling the inside of the walls. Interior panels can either be of fairly basic wood that will be papered over, or fancy panelling, such as oak, that will be left bare and make a modest property look like a stately home. Whatever panelling you use, and the latter is going to be more expensive, a layer of insulating material should be placed between the panels and the solid wall. This, again, is an expensive exercise and requires advice from professionals.

THE ART OF GRACIOUS LIVING

It may be difficult, but keeping your home clear of clutter is the first step to making your home comfortable. When I first set up home on my own I had so many bits of ill-assorted furniture that various friends and relatives had given me, it was difficult to imagine ever having a beautiful home. What with piles of ironing (this was my disorganised period), mountains of books (I refuse to be parted from them), and various bits of bric-à-brac, my flat always looked like a junkyard.

Hoarding things is the main problem. Regularly throw out old magazines – give them to your dentist's or doctor's surgery or the local paper collection. Weed out some of your books occasionally and give them to jumble sales or charity shops. In my first flat I had a very large cupboard that was always filled with things I could never find a use for, or I had forgotten about. When one day I tidied up and cleared out this cupboard, I realised that I had ignored everything in it for over a year. I filled up cardboard boxes with its contents and took them down to the local charity shop. For a while I adopted the practice of putting things away in cupboards until I was in a mood to be ruthless, but now I have advanced to instant ruthlessness.

Ridding yourself of clutter does not mean just organising things into tidy piles. It means either being properly rid of them or putting them in or on something – like shelves. Shelves are cheap to buy and easy to erect. Once all your books and ornaments are on shelves there will be much more floor space.

If you do not have an airing cupboard or somewhere useful to hide all the ironing while you are steeling yourself to do it, then buy an ottoman. I have several such boxes. I have one in the bathroom for dirty washing, which doubles as a seat; I have one in my bedroom for ironing and one in the other bedroom that holds all my sewing materials. I also have one in the corner of the living room that holds all the dog's toys and blankets. The marvellous thing about basic cheap ottomans is that you can paint them any colour to match the prevailing décor of the room and you can cover the lid with padded material, or even carpet, to make a seat.

Wicker baskets or cabin trunks are good too, although rather more expensive.

Furniture

Few of us can afford rooms full of new furniture, even if we wanted it! Often we have a collection of furniture that may not quite match or may have seen better days. A bottle of scratch polish can be a great start to giving old furniture a facelift. Then attacking the soft furnishings is the cheapest way of giving some co-ordination and colour to your home. Nice curtains and matching scatter cushions do wonders for a jaded living room. An old sofa can be covered with a throwover piece of material, meaning that you need not go to the expense of re-upholstery or even stretch or loose covers.

An old dining table can be transformed by a beautiful tablecloth, and old dining chairs can be perked up by attaching seat cushions that match the colour of the tablecloth. You can totally rejuvenate a dining table and chairs bought from a junk shop by painting with emulsion paint and stencilling pretty designs (you can buy templates for this), then varnishing over the finished work.

Feeling good about your surroundings is the best way to feel good about yourself and it doesn't have to cost very much.

Plants

Personally, I could not live without plants. They create such a wonderful display, add life and colour to a room, and it is a joy to nurture them. But then I love growing plants. If you would rather not grow your own, or you do not have time to look after them, you could do worse than invest in artificial plants, some of which are quite stunningly attractive nowadays. I have one, a huge weeping fig which dominates a very dark corner of one room, where a real plant would not flourish. It looks most impressive. It was rather expensive but it will last a lifetime and only needs the occasional spongeing down. Dried flowers are another trouble-free splash of nature in a room.

Decorating

The aim is for bright and cheerful surroundings. Everything you do when you live alone should be part of a plan to make you feel good and ward off depression. There is nothing more depressing than sitting and watching paper peel off the walls. Decorating is cheap and good therapy too.

If you are elderly or disabled, your local Council of Voluntary Service should be able to provide you with willing volunteers to come and decorate for you. Or you could do what my elderly neighbour does: every time she feels like giving her home a facelift, she pays a friend's student son to come and do it for her. Keep it simple if you are on a budget. A few cans of emulsion can do wonders.

There is no point in painting over dirt, though. Keeping your home clean will imbue you with a sense of pride and virtue, which will reflect positively in your own mood. It is difficult to find the time when you are at work all week and it is not much fun spending your only free time cleaning. So, if you have a reasonable income, why not pay someone to do it? If you are elderly or disabled you can organise housework to be part of your care package through your local Social Services.

If you are living on a low income, try this ruse a friend of mine developed when she was young and impoverished. She used to invite people to 'cleaning parties' once a month. Everyone had to bring a cloth, bucket and duster and she guaranteed to provide a few large bottles of cheap wine and a cheap and cheerful meal like a curry or paella. They were great fun. I held a painting party once. I had a huge living room that needed repainting and so I invited a few friends along, asked them to bring a paintbrush each and I supplied the food and drink. We did the room in one day and had fun doing it.

Indulge Yourself

Comfort also means indulgence. No matter how small the treat, or labour-saving device you are able to afford, it is the principle of spoiling yourself that is important. You must always create things to look forward to, to enjoy, and you must always reward yourself each week. It may just be with a cream cake and a magazine, but you are giving yourself a pat on the back. If you love yourself, you will love your own company all the more. Neglect yourself and self-doubt begins to creep in – and that can swiftly turn to depression.

When you have cleaned, polished, decorated and made yourself warm and cosy, you are entitled to treat yourself. If you want to spend your Sunday curled up on the sofa, watching television and having a few drinks, why not? You do not have to worry about anyone else.

Because you live alone, you can devote yourself to making your life easier whenever possible. You cannot spend all your time cooking and cleaning and working. If you can afford it, buy some labour-saving devices, like a washing machine and a tumble drier. Launderettes are fast disappearing anyway and you do not want to spend all your time hand washing and then, in the winter, having clothes hanging all over your home to dry. I bought my first washing machine through an advertisement in the local paper. The machine gave good service for just over a year and then I bought my next one on interest-free credit.

I could not live without a slow-cooker, a steam iron, an electric kettle or a microwave oven. These are the sort of things that you might suggest that people give you as presents, or contribute towards them. I got my food processor and my juice extractor that way.

Televisions, radios and stereo systems bring untold pleasure to countless numbers of people who live alone. I have to confess that I saved up for a portable television before I saved up for a washing machine, but then my priorities may have been different if I had not had a launderette opposite my front door! Of course, buying a television means that you have to buy a licence as well. Buying weekly TV licence stamps can spread the burden somewhat or you can arrange to pay by direct debit if you prefer and certain elderly or disabled people are able to receive help from the local authority with the cost of a licence. Sheltered accomodation units usually purchase one licence for the whole community.

SECURITY

A secure home gives you peace of mind and can be achieved with a little organisation and without any great expense. It will banish any anxieties that you may have about being alone at night or coming home to an empty house.

This section of the book is not meant to frighten you or to cause anxieties. It is intended to make you aware of possible security risks, so that you will feel secure in the knowledge that you have taken all possible precautions. Life today presents many threats to personal security and any woman living alone must take extra care.

Personal Safety

To ensure your own safety at all times, follow these few simple rules:

Close all windows and lock them when you go out. The same goes for doors, of course.

Never open the front door to a caller unless you know the person. If anyone claims to be from the gas or electricity company, the council or any other such body, keep a chain on the door and tell them that you only admit such people by appointment. You have that right. Many people have been tricked by people with false identity cards. Anyway, do you know what a gas company ID should look like? The essential services have no statutory right of entry unless there is an emergency. They can quite easily send you a postcard telling you that a meter inspector will call. Or they can give you a telephone number and wait on the front doorstep while you telephone and check that they are who they claim to be. Do not even admit anyone claiming to be a policeman or woman. Again, do you know all the correct details of a uniform and police ID? The police have no right of entry without a warrant and will certainly understand if you explain politely that you are reluctant to let them in. At the time of writing, British Gas has created a 'personal password' scheme, whereby you can select a personal password, which is known only to you and the gas company. When an engineer comes to call, he has to give that personal password so that you can be reassured he is who he says he is.

When you answer the phone, just say 'Hello' and do not automatically give your name and number.

Ask to have your telephone number made ex-directory if it is not already unlisted. It is quite easy to do this.

Never tell local shopkeepers that you are going on holiday, or announce the fact in a public place. If you need to cancel a delivery, then do so in a note. You never know who may be listening.

Never announce to the world that you have gone away by forgetting to cancel the milk and newspapers. Ask a neighbour to collect your post, water your plants and perhaps to draw your curtains every night and open them each morning. Fit an automatic time switch on your lighting, so that the lights, or perhaps a radio or TV, will switch on and off at night, as though you were there.

Never announce to a group of strangers or in a crowded public place that you live alone. Someone could follow you home after overhearing your conversation.

If you lose your keys, or someone steals your keys, or if you move into a new home and you do not know who may have spare keys, change all the locks immediately.

Phone the police if you see anyone whom you regard as suspicious loitering around outside your home.

Property Risks

Have a good look at your home from outside.

Does the front garden provide good cover for a burglar to work on your windows unseen from the road? You may need to chop down some of those large bushes.

Is your house detached and secluded? This is a magnet to burglars and you need to take all the precautions you can to control access.

Is your back garden secluded and not overlooked by any other property and thus provides another unseen point of entry for a burglar?

Do you have a flat roof at the rear of the house that could provide easy access to upstairs windows? If so, there is nothing you can do about the roof itself but you could have locks put on all your rear windows and replace the glass in them with safety glass (it has a fine wire mesh running through it) which cannot be cut or broken.

Do you have solid iron downpipes that could be climbed? Plastic piping is less popular with burglars.

Do you have an enclosed unlit porch that would give a burglar some cover while working on your door lock? Have a security light fitted, so that the moment anyone walks up to your front door, the light automatically comes on. Or, if you have a porch light, always make sure that it is left on when you are out of the house.

Do you have double-glazed windows? Secondary double glazing adds to the security. Replacement double-glazed units should be chosen to make sure they are safe.

Do you have more than one lock on the front door, bolts, a safety chain, a view-hole and/or entry phone? Despite everything, a lot of burglaries are still carried out via the front door. An ordinary lock can be bypassed with a strip of plastic. You need a deadlock to back it up.

Does your house have a side access? There are several things you can do to make this less vulnerable. Firstly install a lockable, high gate, with metal points on the top to make it difficult to climb over. Secondly, lay down a gravel path around the front of your house and down the side. Burglars hate scrunchy gravel – it's so noisy! Thirdly, install an automatic security light as I mentioned before.

Does your garden back on to an alley or a road? You want tall fencing, lots of spiky, painful bushes in front of them and that security light again.

Does your flat have a balcony or a roof garden? Make it into a really well-stocked garden with lots and lots of potted plants that can be knocked over by intruders trying to climb in.

Does your flat, conservatory or utility room have a skylight in the roof? Fit a lock on such a window and install unbreakable glass.

Do you keep a ladder in your garden shed or greenhouse? If so, it should certainly never be left out in the garden for the convenience of a burglar. The contents of garden sheds are very attractive to burglars – particularly expensive electrical items like mowers, strimmers, etc. So always lock your garden shed and preferably have a proper lock put in the door – padlocks are too easily forced off. Inside the shed, chain all your valuable items to the wall. This is easily done by fixing a metal rail to the shed wall (such as the sort of rail that is used as an aid for disabled people to get out of the bath) then attaching a chain and padlock (the type used to attach bicycles to railings) to the garden equipment and the rail.

Do you have evidence of an alarm system on the outside wall of the house? Even an unwired alarm box is often sufficient to deter a burglar.

Are all your expensive goods easily seen from the front windows? You may think that net curtains are bourgeois but they do hide all your valuables from view. It is a big mistake to have a computer/television/stereo system displayed for all to see from the street.

Are you part of a Neighbourhood Watch Scheme? If so, make sure you display stickers attesting to the fact.

Do you have a dog? They are still the greatest known intruder deterrent.

Do you leave spare keys in hiding places outside the house? Don't – you would be suprised at how good burglars are at finding them. It is much safer to keep your spare key with a trustworthy neighbour. Do not leave keys under the door mat, under potted plants by the front door or hanging on a string inside the letterbox, not even on key racks inside the house. If a burglar breaks into your home through a window, he will want to open the front door to take the television or any other large item out. Don't make it easy for him; double lock the front door and take the keys with you so that he will not be able to open it from the inside.

Do you have glass panels in your front and back doors? Not a good idea if you live alone. Have solid doors. Really solid doors.

Do you have patio doors? These provide the easiest place for a burglar to gain access to a property. They need to have good locks and be fitted with unbreakable glass. If you have inherited patio doors from the previous owner and it would be too expensive to replace them, you might consider having a sliding grille fitted behind the doors, which can be pulled across and locked when you are out.

Do you have decorative walls around your garden? Decorative projecting bricks, wrought iron and other fancy walls and fences provide footholds for intruders to use when they climb into your garden.

Do you have all your valuables, including your car, security marked? There are firms that etch your car windows with serial numbers so that they are more easily traced if stolen. The presence of a security number may deter a car thief because they will have to go to the bother of replacing the windows, which is not an easy job. Precious items of furniture, porcelain, pictures, etc. can be marked with a special invisible pen. Just write on your initials and post code. Then if they are stolen they can be traced and returned to you.

And speaking of cars …

Do you have a removable car radio and cassette/CD player in your car? Very often, thieves will just smash a car window and rip out a car radio. If you have one that can be taken out when you leave the car, it removes that temptation. There are makes of car now which have radios that are impossible to to use without a special code; if yours is one of these, make sure you display a sign saying so and then you won't have your car windows smashed for nothing. Never, of course, leave inviting items visible in the car, such as bags, briefcases, sports gear, etc.

Do you have a car alarm? They do have a value but I am reluctant to recommend these as they can be so temperamental and a public nuisance, if your car is parked in the street. Some of them are set off by the vibration of a passing lorry or by a dog brushing against them and you do not want to keep rushing out in the middle of the night to turn it off. However, if your car is parked in your front garden or in a garage, a car alarm would probably only be set off if the car was being tampered with.

No one is suggesting that you make your home into Fort Knox but a little thought about the above points might help you make it considerably more secure. And the knowledge of that security will give you more peace of mind.

Personal Safety inside the Home

The biggest hazard in the home is fire. Earlier in the book I spoke about making sure you have adequate escape routes in the event of fire; now we will talk about fire prevention. Good internal doors, which are well fitting and should be kept closed as much as possible, can halt a fire by up to 20 minutes, allowing you time to escape.

The kitchen, of course, is the prime source of home fires but there are some guidelines to avoiding disaster:

- Never leave pans that are cooking, particularly frying pans or chip pans. Turn them off and remove them from the heat source if you have to answer the door or the phone.

- Never hang oven gloves or teatowels over cookers.

- Remove polystyrene tiles from the kitchen ceiling. They burst into flames and melt, dropping red hot liquid on to anything that is below, and burning polystyrene also gives off toxic gases.

- Do not keep aerosol containers anywhere near a cooker or source of heat.

- Do not have free-standing oil or paraffin heaters in the kitchen – you could knock them over.

- Make sure that there is always adequate ventilation in a kitchen when cooking, to prevent heat from the oven building up in a confined space.

- Keep a proper fire blanket in the kitchen to be used for smothering fat fires. A fire extinguisher or water should not be used on fat fires.

❧ Do not have loose rugs in the kitchen that you might trip over when holding a hot pan in your hand.

Heating is another danger area but, here too, you can take preventative steps:

❧ Open fires should always have a fire guard – to stop you falling on to the fire if you should trip or stumble.

❧ Open fires should always have the chimney swept regularly, otherwise the build-up of soot and tar can start a chimney fire.

❧ Never hang clothes on a dryer in front of an open fire or a bar heater. One spark and your week's washing could start a conflagration.

❧ Never stand at an open fire warming your back. A spark can just as easily set fire to your clothes.

❧ Do not keep flammable items, such as candles, matches, cigarette lighters, etc. on the mantelpiece or on low tables in front of an open fire.

❧ Make sure that you do not have newspapers or magazines in a pile beside the fire or on top of portable heaters.

❧ Always put out an open fire before going to bed.

❧ Do not put fluffy rugs in front of open fires, where they are in the direct line of sparks.

❧ If you have an open fire in a room, try to have bare floorboards or pure wool, hessian-backed carpets. If you have synthetic or rubber-backed carpets you are in danger from toxic fumes if a fire should start.

- Do not try to draw up an open fire with a sheet of newspaper. It could catch fire in your hands.

- Do not throw rubbish on an open fire in the living room. Many packaging materials contain highly flammable substances which could make a fire suddenly flare up. Also you may throw something on a fire that could give off toxic fumes.

- Make sure that any portable heaters are stable and (particularly in the case of bottled gas or paraffin) that you have adequate ventilation in the room.

- Do not have electric bar fires in the house if you are unsteady on your feet. You should only have wall radiators in your home if that is the case and, if possible, the ones that do not get hot to the touch.

Apart from being careful with sources of heat in your home, there are general preventative measures you can take to avoid the danger of fire.

Do not buy foam-filled furniture if you can avoid it, as it can give off lethal fumes if it ignites. Modern furniture should, by law, be fireproof but your budget may dictate that you buy second-hand. Be careful when choosing. Wooden-framed furniture is best, then at least you can change the cushions for less flammable material.

Ensure that all your gas appliances are regularly serviced. If you suspect a gas leak at any time, do not strike a match or even turn on the electric light, as that can produce a minute spark that can cause an explosion.

Safety with electricity means never operating anything that has a worn or damaged flex; never trying to run an appliance from a light socket; never trying to run too many appliances on an adaptor in one socket; and ensuring that all plugs are wired properly. If you have a power cut, try to switch everything off, except perhaps one light, in case the power comes back on while you are out or asleep.

Beware of cigarettes and never smoke in bed. Never leave a smoking cigarette end in an ashtray. Never empty ashes into cane or rush wastepaper baskets.

The Fire Service recommends that people install smoke detectors in their homes. These are suitable for every room and are cheap and easy to install. They do need to be tested at monthly intervals to ensure that the batteries are still active.

Fire extinguishers are a good idea, but you must be sure to use the right type for each different sort of fire; you could escalate a fire rather than killing it, by using the wrong type of extinguisher. Water can be used to douse any kind of fire except a fat fire or a fire involving electrical equipment. A fire blanket is the simplest option of all and the best thing to have in your kitchen.

ACCIDENTS

The home can be a hazardous place, whether you are young or old, and any sort of accident somehow seems worse when you are on your own. There are several accident blackspots in the home. Take the time to look around your home to identify them. Prevention is always much simpler in the long run than cure.

Floors

Wherever there is water or liquid, there is the danger of it ending up on the floor and causing you to slip. The best thing to do is to put down absorbent floor covering in those rooms. Do not, however, put down loose rugs; they are guaranteed to trip you up. A washable fitted carpet is best in the bathroom, or well-fitting washable carpet tiles, with a backing material that prevents them from creeping. Washable carpet tiles are a good idea in the kitchen, too. It is a very simple matter then to lift and scrub the tiles that take the most punishment, like the ones by the cooker. The value of absorbent flooring is that anything spilt, such as cooking oil (highly dangerous underfoot) immediately disappears instead of lying there, waiting to send you sliding.

Kitchens

Arrange your kitchen so that the sink is very close to the cooker. Many scalding accidents occur when people move from the cooker to the sink to drain off boiling vegetables and either trip or stumble.

Never leave objects on the floor of the kitchen, such as shoes or dustpans, that may trip you up when you back away from the cooker. Shut pets out of the kitchen when you are cooking so that they do not get under your feet.

Do not pile saucepans up higgledy-piggledy on a high shelf, where they can easily fall on top of you when you reach up for something. You should not have anything too high in your house anyway. Many accidents are caused by standing on chairs or stools to reach something and losing balance.

Do not keep sharp knives loose in a drawer. Hang them up or put them in a knife block. You could easily put your hand in a drawer and get hold of the wrong end of a knife.

Be careful when opening tins. Many a hand has come to grief on those lethal corned beef tins or the bare edges of opened tins.

Always observe the sell-by dates on pre-packaged foods and store your food properly. The trouble with living alone is that, sometimes, there are a lot of left-overs which can linger about too long in a fridge and breed nasty things.

Bathrooms

In the bathroom, put a non-slip mat or stickers in the bottom of the bath. Slipping and injuring yourself in the bath is not only painful but can be very serious. If you knock yourself out, you could slip under the water and drown.

Do not have a bath when you are very tired, as you could fall asleep and slip under the water.

Do not put shelves or bathroom cabinets immediately above the washbasin. A friend of mine concussed himself by bending over to splash his face in the basin and cracking his head on a cabinet as he straightened up. Have a plain mirror above the basin and cabinets or shelves elsewhere.

Never take electrical appliances into the bathroom. It is simply not safe to have radios on the side of the bath or electrical heaters plugged into the bathroom in winter, or to use an electric razor in the bath. The combination of water and electricity means instant death – not just a mild shock. In fact, all power points are illegal in bathrooms, except small razor sockets. If you do not have a heated bathroom, then invest in a wall-mounted heater. This must be the type approved for bathroom use, and should be connected through the wall to a power source outside the bathroom. Otherwise you could invest in a thermal light bulb – they throw out a lot of heat. A free-standing oil- or water-filled radiator is all right too, providing, again, the power source is outside the bathroom. But never, never an open bar fire.

Any major appliance in the bathroom such as a washing machine or tumble drier, should always have a properly routed power source outside the bathroom itself. In other words, the cable should be taken through a hole in the wall to the hallway or bedroom; never trail a cable through the bathroom door.

Do not sit in the hottest bath you can stand because this can make you feel faint and you could pass out when you stand up. Similarly, do not have a hot bath after a heavy meal or after drinking alcohol.

Stairs

In the previous chapter I urged you to pick a property where the stairs are of adequate width (this means preferably wide enough for two people to pass) and well-lit, with no awkward corners, no sudden changes in stair depth and with good handrails or bannisters. Make sure that stair carpets are secure and there are no loose treads or worn pieces.

Treat stairs with respect if you want to avoid accidents. Do not put piles of books or magazines up the sides of the stairs. Do not attempt to carry something up or down the stairs that is heavy or awkward or that restricts your visionso that you cannot see where you are placing your feet. Do not leave objects on the stairs.

Do not wear mule-type slippers or flip-flop sandals when going up and down stairs. Do not attempt to wear glamorous stiletto shoes to traverse staircases.

Gardens

In the garden, never leave tools lying around in the grass, particularly rakes or shears that can impale you. Make sure that all sharp implements, such as scythes, have covers, and hang all your tools up, never just throw them into the shed in a muddle – plunging your hand into a pile of assorted implements can be hazardous. Do not keep flammable substances, such as bottled gas or paraffin, in a greenhouse where they are likely to become overheated. Be careful with toxic substances; always follow the directions on the bottle with great care and never decant them into unmarked containers.

Rubbish Disposal

When putting out rubbish, make sure that you wrap broken glass or china in several layers of newspaper to prevent you or the dustmen from being cut. Be careful of old fluorescent light tubes, which can explode when dropped, and never puncture old aerosol cans or throw them on the fire.

Always tie up rubbish bags properly and do not put food on a compost heap – it will only encourage rats and other vermin.

General Points

Being safe in the house is largely a question of organisation and common sense. Give your full concentration to those tasks that you do undertake. A moment's absentmindedness is the cause of many accidents in the home.

- Around the house, generally, do not allow electrical flexes to trail over the floor where you can trip over them.

- Make sure that tall, free-standing items of furniture, like bookcases, are stable and keep heavy items nearer the floor or they will be top-heavy.

- Do not stand on chairs, stools, or steps to reach something at ceiling level unless you have someone with you.

- Bend at the knees to pick up a bulky object, thus avoiding back strain. Get someone to help you with heavy items.

- Don't undertake any job that you really don't feel confident you can accomplish and could possibly be dangerous.

If you are a woman who is classified as being 'at risk', that is, elderly, frail or disabled in some way, then you should seriously consider either living in a sheltered housing complex where you have the safety net of alarms in every room, rigged to a 24-hour warden service, or subscribing to a 24-hour medical alert system. The latter is either a private network, or one set up by the local authority in your area which operates an alarm system at a central control point. Alarms can either be set up in every room in your home or, more usually, you can wear an alarm unit on your person, to activate in times of need. If you want to find out what is available in your area, ask the social services department.

Always leave a key with a neighbour whom you trust and who is at home quite often – maybe someone who is retired or at home with children – in case there is an emergency while you are out and someone needs to get into your house. The real value of a key deposited with your neighbour comes when you are ill or incapacitated and can only call for help or reach the phone, but not reach the front door.

Have a telephone on every floor of your house, if you can. A friend of mine once broke her ankle by falling over in the bathroom and, while she could have dragged herself quite easily along the floor to a telephone in the bedroom if she had had one, as it was, it took her the best part of an agonising hour to struggle down the stairs to the phone in the living room. Extension units need not be too expensive and can be installed by a home handyman. Shop around for prices as it can be more expensive if the telephone company fit the extension.

Eating For One – or More

*F*ood is all things to all people. It can be a comfort, it can be a creative outlet, it can be a source of pride, it can be a pleasure, but most of all it should be the foundation stone of your health.

Just because you live alone is no excuse to not bother to cook. If you always eat out, or live out of tins, you are missing a whole activity of self-fulfilment in life. You can entertain others cheaply and impressively if you bother to cook properly. A friend of mine spends her whole time, now that she is retired, experimenting with different recipes. Every letter I receive from her contains a recommendation to try this or that recipe.

Of course, it can be difficult, when you work or study all day, to arrive home at about seven o'clock and try to feel enthusiastic about preparing a meal. In the same way, if you are elderly and living alone, it may seem like too much bother to cook for yourself. And for disabled people, too, cooking can be such an effort of organisation that they are sometimes tempted not to do anything.

As I have said, though, when you live alone, two things

are very important – firstly, that you love and take care of yourself and, secondly, that you give yourself a treat now and then. Even if you only cook properly at weekends, it is something, and you must not neglect your health by eating processed foods all the time or by skipping meals.

Although there are some marvellous cookery books for single people, I have always found that the trick is not to cook for one, but to cook for four, or whatever the recipe you are following suggests, and to freeze the rest for further meals. That way, you only make the effort to prepare and cook a meal once, and for the other three meals, you just pull something out of the freezer and heat it up. Therefore, good cook books that give freezer recipes are the best idea.

Good utensils can make a real difference to your enjoyment of cooking. Pans which always stick, blunt knives which won't slice properly, frying pans which spit fat in your eye and make your food black because of the carbon deposit build-up, tin openers which don't open tins effectively – they are all guaranteed to put you off cooking altogether.

STORING FOOD

There are lots of ways of storing food and you should try to keep a good variety of items stocked ready in your home. Shopping little and often is expensive and makes no allowance for emergencies.

The Freezer

There is no need to have an enormous freezer, in fact it is better if you do not, unless you grow a lot of garden produce. A small freezer attached to a fridge will serve your needs and be more economical.

A freezer will help you save money, providing you do not keep filling it with expensive exotic ice creams or whole sides of beef. A freezer should be there for you to maximize on your budget by storing cheap and wholesome prepared food, such as soups and stews, and for storing either your own garden produce or purchases of fruit and vegetables when they are at their cheapest. The trick is to buy and cook in bulk and to freeze in small, individual portions. The other advantages of a freezer are that:

- It enables you to store food that can be brought out when you have unexpected guests.

- It enables you to store certain foods in bulk, such as bread, to save you frequent trips to the shops.

- It enables you to prepare food for a dinner party or special occasion well in advance, freeze it, and then have minimal hassle on the day of the party because all you have to do is thaw it out and reheat, cook, or decorate.

- It enables you, as a person who lives alone, to be able to eat foods, such as joints of beef, that you would not ordinarily buy if you did not have some method of storing the left-overs for a considerable period.

Freezing Food

There are plenty of books available on the subject of freezing. Choose one which lists clearly the freezer life of different foods. It should also give you good advice on how to freeze and pack raw and cooked food.

Even if you simply fill your freezer with packaged ready-made meals, at least you are bothering to eat properly and that is important when you live on your own. With a little time and organisation you can eat well and stay healthy.

Your Store Cupboard

There are many methods of storing food over a long period of time, such as preserving, drying and bottling. Jam-making is very easy if you have the right equipment. Save small jars for your jam, and get friends to do the same for you. Large jars are of no use to you if you live on your own – the jam will go mouldy in the opened jar, before you have had a chance to use it up. The sort of small jars that hold olives, mustard, etc. are an excellent size. Be sure to sterilise them thoroughly first though, to remove all taste and smell of vinegar, brine or mustard!

Making your own pickles, chutneys and relishes is definitely worth doing, if you have the time. They have the advantage of keeping well after the jars are opened, so you can use larger jars for these.

It is very easy to dry your own herbs. Spread the herbs out on trays covered in sheets of paper and place them in an airing cupboard or other warm, dry place for about five to seven days. Turn them over every day and the plants are ready when the leaves are brittle and crumble between the fingers. Store them in airtight containers, preferably away from strong light. There are several good books that give comprehensive advice on growing and storing herbs.

Bottling fruit in the summer and autumn, when there is a glut, is a wonderful way of preserving fruit for use in wintertime. It is possible to buy small Kilner jars (0.5 litre), which hold just enough plums, apricots, sliced apples, etc. in syrup for one person to eat, perhaps at two meals. Or you could bottle up a few larger jars of fruit, for use in pies and crumbles when you have guests.

Two storage items that are really useful are a brine crock and a rumtopf (or rumpot). A brine crock is great for storing runner beans for a long time. What you need is a wide-necked earthenware container – something like a bread crock. You then put layer after layer of washed, fresh runner beans and plenty of salt in the container, put the lid on, or cover the top with a cloth and put it in a cool, dark place. After a while, the salt and the moisture from the beans forms a powerful brine, that perfectly preserves the beans. Whenever you want some, you just grab a handful out of the crock, wash them thoroughly, and you have delicious beans ready for cooking.

A rumtopf is the same sort of thing, in other words an earthenware container, but its purpose is to preserve soft fruits in alcohol. Quite simply, you put layer after layer of any fruits into the container, after they have been left overnight soaking up a certain quantity of sugar, then you submerge each layer of fruit in rum or brandy. You have to stir it thoroughly quite often, otherwise the sugar gets sludgy. After about three months you have an extremely powerful, alcoholic mixture which tastes heavenly. It must be used in small doses, however, such as spooned over some ice cream or nestling beside some biscuits. Be careful if you or your guests are driving!

A well-stocked storage cupboard, combined with a freezer, should see you through any emergency brought about by weather or illness. Replacing every item as you use it is a sure way of always being prepared – and of being certain what you have in your store cupboard.

I store most things in see-through glass jars, which makes it easier to see at a glance what I have in stock. Also, leaving some foods in their opened packets, shortens their storage life. Much better to keep them in air-tight jars.

BUYING FRESH PRODUCE

There is little to say about this except that if living alone is a new experience for you, you will tend to buy too much at first and waste a lot, unless you cook and freeze. If you can't do that, then the way to guard against waste is to buy little and often. I have found that it is a mistake to buy fresh food once a week: I either run out of organisational steam halfway through the week, so all the meals I have planned to cook fall by the wayside, or I get held up at work or in some other way, and end up grabbing fish and chips on the way home instead. In any event, half the food bought at the weekend is wasted.

If you are unused to living alone you may also find that you cook too much food. Try to discipline yourself to using up left-overs. I have a dog, which helps. She is happy to eat left-over mashed potato and positively loves cold rice pudding!

I often use up left-over vegetables in a Spanish omelette or as part of a rice-based meal, a sort of risotto. That is why rice and pasta are such useful things to have in the store cupboard, because you can mix them with anything. A plate of pasta, mixed with fried courgettes and some mushrooms covered with a packet cheese sauce, takes only 15 minutes to prepare.

USEFUL COOKING AIDS

Try to aim for a small collection of really good cooking aids – ask for them as Christmas presents or collect petrol tokens. If possible, buy things which have a double use – oven to tablewear, for example, or a pan whose lid doubles as another serving dish.

Slow-cookers: These are wonderful – I would not be without mine.

A slow-cooker is an earthenware pot, with a lid, set in a metal frame which contains a heating element. They come in various sizes. I now have two. I use one for savoury dishes and one for sweet dishes, mainly because I use my savoury one a lot and if you cook lots of curries, the taste can linger a bit in the earthenware.

Everything cooks very slowly in a slow-cooker because the heating element is extremely low-powered and costs no more to use than leaving a light bulb switched on for a day (a few pence). You can fill it up with all the ingredients necessary for your soup, stew, casserole or pudding, switch it on before you go out in the morning, and you will arrive home to a wonderful smell and a meal that is ready to serve. Slow-cookers make meat beautifully tender (you can roast a joint and it will not shrink as it might in the dry heat of the normal oven) and they cook perfect custards and sauces. Most dishes take eight to ten hours to cook, so some ingredients, such as pasta, should be added later in the process, otherwise they disintegrate.

A good slow-cooker will come with a recipe book, but there are many recipe books that deal specifically with slow-cooking, now available at booksellers.

Food Processors: These take all the effort out of preparing food, as they do all the chopping, slicing, grating, blending, whisking and kneading incredibly fast. The only disadvantage I find with them is that there are so many bits to take apart and wash and, as with most plastic bowls, it is difficult to rid them of the smell of onions. In an ideal world I suppose one should have two – a sweet and a savoury – like my slow-cookers, but that is rather extravagant.

Blenders: Very useful, particularly if you make nourishing soups in your slow-cooker and you occasionally want to purée them.

Juice Extractors: A good idea for people living alone because they enable you to juice one orange at a time, when you fancy some juice, whereas a litre carton may well start fermenting before one person can drink it all.

Microwaves: Microwaves have been adopted by busy people up and down the country. They are a boon if you have a hectic lifestyle. If you are busy or infirm, the advantage of being able to take a ready-made meal out of the freezer and put it in the microwave where it can defrost and cook in under 15 minutes, far outweighs any aesthetic pleasure that purists might derive from lengthy cooking processes. Microwaves are also very economical for the single person. Unlike conventional ovens, the less you put into them, the less time it takes to cook.

Finally, especially if you are living alone for the first time, invest in some small cooking dishes and fridge/freezer containers. That way you can cook and store the right amounts for a meal for one person. You will, of course, need some larger dishes and containers for when you entertain guests.

ECONOMICAL ENTERTAINMENT

Entertaining friends need not be expensive or difficult. Your biggest investment should be your time in preparation for the event.

There is no reason why single women should not entertain and give dinner parties, and yet the very idea of it is enough to put some of us off. There are, it's true, lots of pitfalls in formal entertaining but if you are nervous about giving proper dinner parties, then don't – there are plenty of other ways to entertain your friends. Forget seating plans and balancing numbers – people are much less stuffy these days and your friends will probably welcome the chance just to join you for an informal supper.

Guests Who Come to Stay

If a friend descends upon you unexpectedly, you just have to hope that whatever you have in the freezer will suffice. If you do not have a freezer, then you will have to shop during your friend's stay.

However, if you are given advance warning, think about the stay and about the meals you will have to provide. Discuss the question of food and drink. If your visitor has a food allergy then it is best if they bring their special foods with them, as you may not be able to obtain them yourself.

A typical weekend visit where the guest arrives on Friday night and departs on Sunday night will normally mean that you have to cater for two dinners (Friday and Saturday night), two breakfasts (Saturday and Sunday mornings), two lunches (Saturday and Sunday) and one tea (early Sunday evening).

It is best to make it as trouble-free as possible. Firstly, make your Friday night meal a cold one, because your guest may arrive late or you may have to go and meet your guest at the bus or railway station. Just cold meat and salad or something similar, so you don't have to worry. Make sure that you have all the breakfast options available – eggs, bacon, cereal, toast. Make a simple one-pot meal for Saturday evening dinner (like a stew in the slow-cooker, so that you are not forever preparing meals or washing up). A slow-cooker, of course, will allow you and your guest to spend the whole of Saturday out and about, without worrying about the preparation of the meal when you get home.

If you can afford it, eat out modestly once or twice during the stay. Have a pub snack, for instance, on the Saturday when you are out shopping or sightseeing, and a roast lunch on Sunday. Eating out (particularly Sunday lunch) gives you a break from cooking and gives your guest some variety of scenery.

The Dinner or Luncheon Party

Whatever time of day it is, this is most likely to mean inviting a group of people for a 'sit-down' meal. The grandness of the meal, and how much of it you pay for, depends upon the expectations of yourself and your guests and also perhaps their relationship to you.

Most friends, of any age, would bring a bottle of something – unless the dinner party is very grand.

Relatives, however, often seem to feel that they do not need to bring a contribution, unless, of course, you are being visited by your mother, in which case, whatever your age, she will probably bring a month's supply of food and wash up for you as well!

Whether it is lunch or dinner, don't make it too complicated. If the meal is to be three courses, then make the first and last courses cold – seafood cocktail and chocolate mousse, for example – prepare them the night before and put them in the fridge. Do not give yourself a nervous breakdown trying to prepare and cook three courses perfectly on the day. Don't have a rigid timetable, guests are often late and rarely sit down at the table on time. So, if you have a cold starter and a dessert and a main course that is either a one-pot meal, like a casserole or a roast, where the oven temperatures can be adjusted to cope with delays in starting, then you should avoid crises.

Do not believe any articles you read that are written by restaurateurs, chefs or cordon bleu cooks about either soufflés, profiteroles or flambés being the simplest thing in the world. They are recipes for disaster when you are entertaining. You are coping alone – whereas people who cook for a living invariably have an army of helpers contributing towards the perfect meal.

For a really cheap and cheerful gathering of friends you

could do worse than curry, spaghetti bolognese, some kind of fondue or pizza.

If you are going to eat alfresco then I would give you two tips: firstly, make most of the meal cold – it will only get cold between your kitchen and your garden anyway. You could perhaps introduce the odd hot item such as garlic bread, wrapped in tinfoil, to complement a salad, or a hot fudge sauce to pour over an ice cream dessert.

The second tip is that if you are planning an evening meal outside, do not have candles or any kind of light on the dining table itself. Have the lighting some distance away from the table, otherwise all your food, you and your guests, will be covered in moths, mosquitos and midges before you even reach the main course.

Parties

Parties need careful planning and handling when you live alone (see Chapter 8). Again, where food is concerned, the main thing is not to be too ambitious. You cannot answer the door, take people's coats, give people drinks, circulate and generally be a good hostess if you have to keep popping into the kitchen.

Hot food is not feasible unless you have a hot tray, an electric fondue, or a slow-cooker, all of which can be used to keep things warm on a buffet table. Cold food, such as crisps, nuts, sausage rolls, quiches, French bread and cheese, may be rather predictable, but can be easily and quickly topped up. Sandwiches and canapés go stale very quickly at a party. A variety of cheeses and a pâté, French bread and butter are simple and popular. People will help themselves and save you a lot of work, as will buying paper plates for everyone to use.

In general, people prefer finger buffets at stand-up parties anyway, because it is terribly difficult to eat a fork buffet if you can't sit down. Do not forget to provide one or two items of sweet food – individual cakes or petit fours. Very creamy cakes or gateaux are likely to deposit their fillings on your carpet though!

Don't forget that quite a few people are vegetarians nowadays and you must cater for them. I would also counsel against serving seafood such as mussels, cockles, whelks, etc. It is embarrassing, not to mention worrying, if your guests come down with tummy upsets the next day, and seafood is always a bit risky.

Looking After Yourself

You are the only person who can take care of your health. When you do not live with anyone else there is no one to nag you about smoking, drinking, eating too much, eating too little or eating the wrong things. Neither is anyone going to fetch and carry for you when you are in bed with influenza, or be there to patch you up when you fall over, burn yourself or cut yourself. This makes three things essential:

- ఴ That you take the best possible care of yourself to avoid ill-health

- ఴ That you do not become a hypochondriac.

- ఴ That if you do become ill, you accept the fact and do everything possible to recover.

TAKING GOOD CARE OF YOURSELF

Health Promotion

Regular exercise is very important, and the best forms of exercise are walking, swimming, cycling and gardening. If you can, try to do some kind of exercise that makes you breathe hard for about ten minutes each day. This is very good for your heart and lungs. If you are at work all the time and find fitting in regular exercise quite difficult, then invest in an exercise bike or a rowing machine. Ten minutes in the morning should keep you trim. However, do not suddenly take up violent exercise after years of inactivity or you will injure yourself. The ten minutes of hard breathing mentioned above is enough to start with.

Many people like to do exercises to music and there are plenty of options – you can go to classes, devise your own exercises to music, buy one of the hundreds of exercise cassettes and videos available. Do not be too ambitious with exercises: start off with something gentle, that suits all age groups. Reject videos that go for the 'burn' or videos demonstrated by 18-year-olds in minimal Lycra. If the fact that you can't manage the exercises doesn't depress you, the sight of tiny waists and perfect unsupported breasts will have you reaching for the Prozac!

Mental fitness is very important too. You must exercise your mind each day in the same way that you do your body. Think positively every day about what is right with your life. Do not sidetrack into dwelling on what is wrong with it. A psychiatrist I spoke to when researching this book advised a list method. When you wake up, if you feel depressed or lonely, write down all the positive things about your life :

I am in good health

I have a nice house

I have a good job

My dog loves me and I love my dog

The sun is shining today – and so on.

Force yourself to do it, no matter how low you feel. The effort you need to make to think positively is the same as the effort you need to make to force weak leg muscles to ride a bike: it makes you stronger in the end.

Laughter is a marvellous preventative medicine – whether you feel low or not it always does you good to take yourself off to the nearest comedy film or show. Or read a funny book. Or phone up a cheerful friend who always makes you laugh. Go out with that friend. Have a meal out, go shopping – just go out. Go out with other people and just listen to them laugh. One of the great things about watching a good comedy show or film is that the people around you start to laugh and you cannot help joining in. Make the effort to join in the 'fun' things. If there is a local carnival each year, or a firework display, or carol singing – go and enjoy the general festive atmosphere. Singing is a wonderful way to relax and revitalise yourself. Scientists have proved that it does actually release chemicals in the brain that create pleasure and relax you. This is why so many people find going to church a pleasurable experience.

Avoiding Hypochondria

When you live alone it is very easy to magnify every little ache and pain into a life-threatening illness. Having said that, it is far better to make a fool of yourself by going to the doctor with an imagined breast lump, than to ignore what could be a real breast lump. Seeing your health in perspective is the important thing. If you eat the right foods and take some exercise, you will begin to understand and know your body better and you will be able to discern the difference between a muscular ache which has its cause in some action you have taken, and a pain which you have never encountered before.

Do not spend your life taking over-the-counter medication for the slightest ache or pain. Synthetically produced drugs are toxic – even taken in small quantities. Very often a headache or a stomach upset is a sign that your system is polluted anyway – in the same way that a hangover is caused by your system trying to cope with an influx of alcohol – so taking pills or powders for your headache or stomach upset will only add to your system's toxicity. Try drinking lots of water instead, or not eating at all for a day to clear out the toxins (unless you are diabetic or have some other dietary problem); have a warm bath and a nap, or go for a long walk. All these things are just as likely to rid you of a headache as taking a pill.

Avoid taking laxatives. If you eat plenty of fresh fruit and vegetables, drink plenty of liquid and exercise regularly, you should have no need for them. However, if you have been taking laxatives for so long that you are caught up in a chemical spiral and cannot now function without them, then a two-day fast on fruit juice and water will break the cycle. Again, this should only be attempted if your doctor agrees that you are otherwise in good health.

If you are tense then you could try some of the natural relaxant products that are available through health food stores and chemists. There are herbal tranquillisers and sleeping tablets and relaxing herbal teas which can give an excellent night's sleep.

Recognising When You Need Help

For many women alone, there can be frightening times in their lives, often caused by the changes in hormone levels during the menopause, or by the shock of bereavement or divorce. There are times when you have no control, and no matter how hard you try to cope, the panic attacks come for no reason. Bad clinical depression in fact rarely makes people think of suicide, it just gradually envelops your life until everything is coloured grey and you have lost interest in everything that previously made you happy, stimulated or content.

These are the times when you need medical help. But you have to recognise the symptoms for yourself and go and ask the doctor for help. Bad depression can affect your appetite by making you eat more or eat less; it can affect your sleep by either making you unable to sleep or making you want to do nothing but sleep; it can wipe out your desire for sex; it can make you lose interest in yourself and others; it can make you anxious and anti-social; it can make you cry easily or make you introverted and numbed.

If you feel that your personality has changed in some of the ways described above, or friends tell you that you have changed, and you realise that you have lost control of your emotions, then you are most probably depressed and in need of help. Do not try to cope alone. There are times in your life when you have to have medication to get you back on an even keel. You will not be able to conquer it alone and, if left, depression will probably get worse.

Tranquillisers, anti-depressants or sleeping tablets should only be taken if they are really needed. During a bad crisis they may help, but when you are feeling stronger you should stop taking them. GPs nowadays constantly review the length of term of the drugs that they prescribe. No longer are patients left on repeat prescriptions indefinitely. Do not stop long-term medication overnight, however, because it is possible to suffer withdrawal symptoms that panic sufferers into taking the pills for the rest of their lives. Your doctor will help you cut down on them gradually by prescribing progressively weaker doses.

WHEN YOU ARE ILL

Even the healthiest person can succumb to an illness that is prevalent locally. It is very difficult, particularly for those who work in stuffy, overcrowded offices, to which they commute on stuffy, overcrowded trains, to avoid catching a cold or some other virus.

When you catch something like this, the first thing you should do is give in to it. No matter what your business commitments, it is far more sensible to have one day at home in bed to recover from the worst of the virus, than to struggle into work, making yourself ill for longer and giving the virus to everyone else. Some viruses can be so vicious that if you do not take care of yourself for a couple of days when you first fall ill, you could spend three weeks or more feeling under par.

With any virus, going to bed, making yourself as warm as possible, drinking plenty of fruit juice and water (not milk) is the best form of treatment. This will help to eliminate the virus through your sweat and urine as fast as possible. Sleep is a great help to any illness, so sleep as much as you can. Call the doctor in if you want to, but since most viruses are beyond the skills of any doctor he will probably just give you the same advice as above.

Always call the doctor if you have severe vomiting or diarrhoea. In either case you can very quickly dehydrate and put your life at risk. Call the doctor if any part of your body swells up or you come out in spots or rashes.

Making Arrangements for Illness and Convalescence

A key deposited with a trustworthy neighbour and the location of a telephone and address book beside the bed are invaluable at times of illness, because you can call the neighbour and doctor from your sickbed and the neighbour can let the doctor in for you.

If you have to stay long in bed, or at least at home, you will need to make arrangements so that you can cope. Firstly, you will need to make arrangements to get someone to do your shopping, unless your local shop will take an order over the phone and deliver it for you. You will probably need plenty of fruit juices, fruit, soup and possibly a food supplement, such as Complan. Ring your local surgery and ask if they can have your prescriptions delivered.

If you are elderly or disabled, your doctor can probably arrange for the district nurse to visit you to see that you are all right, to give you a bed bath or put on bandages, apply ointment to rashes, etc. If you cannot get shopping delivered and you have other problems, like a dog that needs walking, you could try ringing your local Council for Voluntary Service to see if they can provide a volunteer to pop in and do those things for you.

Emergency Hospitalisation

If you have to be hospitalised then, again, it will be necessary to organise some kind of support. If your hospitalisation is sudden – say you are struck down with appendicitis at work – ask your work colleagues or one of the nurses in the hospital to telephone your neighbour who has the key and ask him or her to check that your home is all right, look after your pet until you can make other arrangements, water your plants and generally keep an eye on things. Alternatively, either colleagues or a neighbour could ring a friend or relative, who might move into your home and take care of things while you are in hospital. Do not worry about things like night clothes and toilet things – the hospital will have everything you need.

Planned Hospitalisation

If your hospital stay is planned, then you will have plenty of time to organise some help to take care of your home and other responsibilities. If you have no family, neighbours or friends available to help, there are businesses that offer 'home- and pet-sitting' services. They will either put someone in your house on a full-time basis, or they will send someone round every day to check on things. Prices will probably vary according to the amount of work they have to do.

Your home will not suffer for a couple of weeks without anyone to look after it any more than it does when you go on holiday. You will have to lodge your pet with someone, if you have one, but most friends or neighbours will happily take a fishtank, caged bird or animal for a week or two, providing you give them written instructions and all the food, bedding and other necessities. Dogs or cats can be boarded at kennels. Plants will survive quite happily if you group them all together in the bath, soak them well, and leave about an inch of water in the bottom of the bath. The humidity created by grouping them together in the bath will keep them moist for quite a while. Just make sure that they are not standing in direct sunlight.

Turn off all the heating and gas (but don't forget to make arrangements to have them turned on prior to your return). Unless it is deep winter, do not turn off the cold water, particularly if you want a neighbour to come in and water plants or run a hose from the kitchen to water the garden. Do not turn off the electricity either. Your neighbour may only be able to visit your house in the evening and will need light. Equally, the electricity may be needed for your alarm system and lights which deter burglars.

Encourage as many people as possible to visit you when you are in hospital. They will help you not to feel isolated or depressed while you are ill and away from home. If you have no one to visit you, then you can tell the nurse that you would be grateful for a hospital visitor. These are part-time volunteers who come and visit any patients who are alone. They will chat, bring you some magazines, and run errands for you. Undoubtedly you will receive a visit from the hospital chaplain. Don't be put off – even if you are not religious, it is a welcome chance for social contact and the exchange of a few pleasantries.

Having an operation naturally entails feelings of anxiety, so talk to as many professional people as you can – doctors, nurses, the anaesthetist when he or she comes to visit you – to reassure yourself. With a planned hospital stay, you will have been told to prepare for the operation as best you can, perhaps by losing some weight, or attempting to stop smoking. All these measures are designed to give you as trouble-free a recovery as possible. You must also try to relax as much as you can. If you are admitted the day before your operation and cannot sleep, tell the nurse and he or she will give you a sleeping pill.

Post-operative and Convalescent Care

After the operation you may feel sick or very depressed – this is the effect of the trauma of the operation and of the anaesthetic and is only temporary. Knowing the cause will help you pull through it, and you will feel better very quickly when the effects of the anaesthetic wear off. Do not try and rush your recovery. Many people leap out of bed and charge about the ward on their first day after the operation, only to collapse in a heap the day after that.

When you are approaching the end of your hospital stay (and they are extremely short nowadays) you will have to think about convalescence at home . Do not underestimate the effect that even a small operation has on your body and your nervous system. An abdominal operation may leave you unable to lift or carry things for at least a month. Back and leg operations may prevent you from walking up any stairs and may even immobilise you completely for a while.

It is necessary to prepare for convalescence before you go into hospital, if that is at all possible. If you genuinely feel that you can cope at home, with the help of neighbours and friends, make sure that you have in plenty of supplies – food, drink, clean nightwear and underwear and so on. That will eliminate the need for shopping, washing and ironing after your return from hospital. Before you go into hospital, put downstairs everything that you will need on your return – the television, the radio, your favourite books, your plants, the paperwork that you are going to catch up on. Ask someone to go in and turn on the heating if it has been turned off in your absence.

You may need to re-arrange your home somewhat. You could have the bed moved downstairs if you live in a house and, if you do not have a downstairs toilet, contact the Red Cross and arrange for the loan of a portable toilet/commode. Your GP will make any necessary arrangements, e.g. the district nurse to come in regularly to change your dressing, help you bath, supervise your medication, etc.

If you are elderly and the operation you are having is quite major, then be realistic. Unless you can arrange for someone to come and stay with you for at least a month, you will not be able to cope. Therefore, you may want to arrange with the hospital for a place in a convalescent home for the post-operative phase. You may have to pay for this facility, but at least you will have the peace of mind of being waited on hand and foot until you are better.

WHAT TO DO IF YOU HAVE AN ACCIDENT

The vast majority of accidents in the home are, thankfully, very minor; for these you should always have a First Aid kit well-stocked and handy. Keep it in the kitchen (the most likely scene of accidents) and, if you live in a house with two or more storeys, keep one on each floor as well. There is little point in having a first aid kit on the ground floor if you cut your foot badly upstairs.

A good first aid box should contain the following:

Several bandages in various sizes, including a crêpe bandage for sprains

A small pair of scissors that will cut in awkward little corners

A roll of cotton wool (not cotton wool balls)

Individually packed sterile dressings in various sizes

A pair of tweezers

Safety pins

Sticking plaster on a roll

Antiseptic lotion and cream

Antihistamine cream

Gauze

Always replace items you have removed or used.

If you have injured yourself badly, for example broken your leg, concussed or burnt yourself, call an ambulance. Dial 999, ask for the ambulance service and state your name and address clearly. If you can manage to go to the front door, open it before you pass out or feel faint, or phone a neighbour who has a key. Then lie or sit down on the nearest piece of furniture, try to keep warm and wait calmly for help to arrive.

Do not drink or eat anything at all. You may need an anaesthetic when you get to hospital, or you could pass out while attempting to eat or drink and choke. Shock affects the blood pressure, so you should neither smoke nor drink alcohol as this would further affect the blood pressure. If you have fractured a bone or fallen on your back, do not move at all, as this could make things worse. If you do not have a personal alarm, or access to an alarm system, then try to shout for help, or bang on the floor or wall.

If you are bleeding badly, then try and stop the flow of blood by pressing on the wound with a large pad of cotton wool, or some clean material. Do not attempt to tie a tourniquet unless you think that you have severed an artery. If you do have to tie a tourniquet, do not keep up the pressure for longer than ten minutes and allow at least one minute between re-applications. As soon as you start to apply a tourniquet, then write on your arm or leg with a pen the time that application started. Do this every time you re-apply the tourniquet. That way, if you should pass out before the ambulance arrives then they will know when you last applied pressure.

In any case of bleeding, sit or lie down and try to raise the affected part of the body so that the blood flows less quickly. If it is not a severe wound that requires the attention of an ambulance crew, and you are fairly mobile, wash the wound before attending to it – unless it was caused by splinters of glass or some other small fragments, which you may push in deeper by touching it. You should go to the casualty department of a hospital to have any wound properly looked at as soon as possible. You will probably have to have an anti-tetanus injection, which prevents any infection, particularly if you have cut yourself while gardening.

If you have a nose bleed, apply pressure to the nose by pinching the nostrils together for about ten minutes. If that does not work, try packing the nostrils with cotton wool and applying ice cubes to either side of the nose.

If you have a chest, head or abdominal wound, keep as still as possible and do not touch the wound. Summon help immediately.

If garden chemicals get on to your skin, plunge the affected part into cold water. If your eyes are affected, plunge your face, with your eyes open, into water. Keep doing this until any pain subsides, then cover the affected area and go to the hospital, taking the bottle of chemicals with you.

If you start to choke on something, put your fist into the soft spot under the middle of your ribcage and press in hard, repeatedly, or bend forward over the back of a chair and bounce your abdomen off it. Both these actions should help force the matter up out of the windpipe. If it does not work, go out into the street and find someone to help.

If you burn or scald yourself, immediately immerse the affected part in cold water for as long as possible, or put a cold wet pad over it. Remove any tight clothing or jewellery because swelling could occur. As with bleeding, raise the affected part, so that circulation slows down. Do not put any cream on the burn, it should be kept dry. Leave blisters alone, just loosely cover everything with a clean cloth and call the doctor or go to the nearest casualty department if you can. If you have burnt your mouth, suck ice in order to stop any swelling occurring that may constrict your airway. You should do the same if you are stung in the mouth by a bee or wasp.

If your clothes catch fire, grab the nearest large cloth – rug, tablecloth, coat – and try to smother the fire. Hold it over yourself tightly and roll in it on the floor. Do not try to remove burnt material that has attached itself to your skin.

If you should faint, when you recover consciousness, do not attempt to do anything other than call the doctor or a neighbour and lie down on the bed.

Hypothermia

Hypothermia is essentially an insidious condition that happens over several hours, with the victim becoming sleepier and sleepier and not realising that she is slowly freezing to death. During periods of cold weather the elderly or disabled are particularly vulnerable because of their lack of mobility, although younger people can suffer from the condition if they become severely chilled. It can occur overnight if the victim has been sleeping in a poorly-heated room with insufficient bedclothes. You can avoid hypothermia by always dressing warmly in several loose layers, keeping the home as warm as possible, taking frequent warm drinks, and moving about as much as possible. Wear warm nightclothes and bedsocks in bed and if the weather is very cold, leave the heating on a low setting overnight.

Anything but Lonely

*I*t can sometimes seem hard to have an active social life if you live by yourself. Of course, not everyone wants to – for some, peace and solitude are sheer heaven. But if you do like the company of other people, entertaining at home is the best way of controlling the scale of your social involvement. This does not mean lavish dinner parties every night – inviting people into your home need be no more than a modest invitation to one person to come and have a cup of coffee and a biscuit.

COMPANY IN YOUR HOME

There are all sorts of opportunities for this. For instance, if you are talking to a neighbour and he or she seems in no particular rush, then invite him or her in for an impromptu cup of something.

Sunday lunchtime is a good opportunity to invite neighbours and friends into your house for a few drinks and tit-bits. It seems to be the most convenient for many people since they do not have to drive in the dark, and they can have a much more leisurely meal without having to worry about the time. Friends who live quite a long way away can come to have Sunday lunch with you, whereas for dinner there would probably not be enough time. Also, Sunday lunches, especially in the summer, are so lovely and relaxed. One can have them outside in the garden, or on a patio or balcony, and the whole day can be stretched to include tea and cakes at around four o'clock. Summer tea parties with scones and strawberries served on the lawn are an appealing and inexpensive way to entertain.

Summer is also a marvellous time to have 'open house' days; these are marvellous opportunities to invite all sorts of people – friends, neighbours, relatives – to visit any time, between, say, eleven o'clock in the morning and ten o'clock at night. A cold buffet, which can be topped up throughout the day, is ideal, and people can float in and out, stopping just for a drink and a few peanuts, or staying much longer. Only those of you with plenty of stamina should attempt an 'open day' however, since a 12 hour stint of entertaining requires forethought and energy. Once a year is probably quite often enough.

Sometimes, the simpler parties are the most successful. I have a friend who holds 'getting to know the neighbours' spaghetti parties. These simply involve inviting a handful of neighbours in for a fairly informal plate-on-your-lap spaghetti meal and a few glasses of wine.

There are lots of excuses for throwing a party: your birthday, a house-warming, a new job, and so on. However, when you live alone and you are inviting comparative strangers to your party, it is wise to enlist the help of a friend beforehand to help you cope. You may also like help with the planning and execution of the catering. Elderly people may turn to a younger relative or friend to help them host a party.

A party, though, can be just a handful of people – you do not have to overstretch your resources or capabilities. I have had some excellent parties of no more than ten people on winter evenings. We have helped ourselves to a buffet, had a few drinks, watched television and even played games.

Whatever the form of your home entertaining, always make sure that you feel in control of it. Make it the sort of occasion that does not cost you a fortune and one that gives you pleasure, not anxiety.

A WORD ABOUT CHRISTMAS AND NEW YEAR

The purpose of this book is to make you enjoy your time living alone. If you are truly alone, then public holidays, particularly Christmas and New Year, can be depressing.

Try to take a positive view: tell yourself that this time, it is going to be different. Personally, I have no fears about spending Christmas Day completely on my own. To me, it is such a wonderful luxury.

Just think. On Christmas morning, you can have a lie-in, then get up and have a luxurious bath with perfume and candles, while listening to some wonderful music. You can dress in whatever makes you feel comfortable and you can eat and drink whatever you want throughout the day. You can curl up by the fire, read a good book, watch what you want to watch on television, or watch a video. You can pamper yourself. If you want some company, you can have a drinks party on Christmas Eve, go to church on Christmas

Day, go to the local pub at lunchtime, or go to a pantomime on Boxing Day.

The secret of an enjoyable solo Christmas is to make the effort just for yourself. Decorate your home with Christmas decorations, have a Christmas tree, buy yourself a few little treats in the month leading up to Christmas and wrap them up to open on Christmas Day. None of this is sad. It is a positive move to put you in the Christmas mood. You don't have to have traditional Christmas dinner, although if you want it, many of the large food retailers now do turkey breast portions that make, at most, three meals for a single person. You can have smoked salmon and caviare, if you want – you don't have to think of anyone else but yourself. It can be wonderful.

If you really cannot bear the thought of Christmas on your own, then you could do what many other single people of all ages do – go on a holiday, where Christmas is taken care of. It could be a country house hotel in the UK, or a place in the sun, but someone else does all the work. All the festivities are laid on and there are even presents dished out for the guests. You meet lots of people in a similar position to yourself and the holiday can be one endless party with the option of escaping to your own room if you want some peace and quiet for a while.

Whatever you do, make sure that you do not get depressed over the whole business of Christmas being for families. I think that it is vastly overrated anyway, and I doubt that it was ever the jolly occasion we have all been brainwashed into expecting.

GOING OUT

Now, forget about Christmas and think about the rest of the year and the possibilities for your social life outside the home. Do not feel that you have to join a group – it may not be what you want.

The first and most important thing in maintaining a social life is that you take the time and make the effort to keep those friends that you already have. Do not say 'Oh I must get round to phoning Fred or Millie' and just keep putting it off. Make regular calls and write regular letters. Keep a note of birthdays in your diary, so that you do not forget to send friends and relatives cards and/or presents. Make the effort to send everyone a Christmas card each year. Do not let friendships lapse. It is very easy to do, especially if friends have moved away and are always busy.

You can bring some variety and social contact into your life by simply going out and talking to people. Instead of merely shopping, take the time to exchange a few words with shop assistants. Go to local jumble sales and bazaars and go to local amateur dramatic performances. Members of such groups are usually very friendly and so grateful that people turn up to their performances that they are quite often there to smile and chat to visitors at the door. Go to your nearest town occasionally for a special event – a concert, a festival, or a flower show. All these things you can do by yourself, but at the same time you will be making some sort of social contact.

You could develop an interest that brings you into contact with other people, like collecting paintings or other objets d'art. Even if your interest only takes you on regular window-shopping tours of your local antique or junk shops, it will give you some stimulation.

There are also ways of developing friends at a distance, like penfriends for example. This is not an activity restricted to schoolchildren, there are lots of organisations who will find penfriends for people of all ages. You may find yourself opening up a whole new world of exciting foreign contacts which could, eventually, lead to some lasting friendships and charming holidays.

Socialising in a Group

Many people find that they enjoy being involved with some sort of club activity and with other members of a group. However, you should only join clubs, societies or associations if the work or activity that they pursue is really of interest to you, or it is unlikely to be a success. I once joined a flower-arranging society, thinking, 'Well I quite like flowers and it's a good way to meet people' but it just was not for me. I found it so boring that I left after a month. I realised that I needed something that was a bit more active and fairly creative, preferably something that included both sexes (I love my own sex dearly, but sometimes the conversation can be almost entirely about babies or, at the other end of life, the menopause!). I now belong to my local drama group, which is great fun, and my local history group, which is fascinating. So look for what suits you. Find out about local organisations and societies at your local library.

Evening classes are a good way of meeting people, adding to your skills, having fun and learning at the same time, without the organisational demands that a club may make upon you. Most classes are advertised in the local press, or at libraries, during the summer months. There is a whole range of classes that start at any time during the year and lots of classes during the day for the early retired.

Of course, the same rule applies to classes as it does to clubs – they must be on a subject that really interests you. Otherwise, after a hard day's work, in the middle of winter, you will find that you cannot be bothered to make the effort to go along.

Do not forget that for the elderly and disabled there are day centres and 'pop-in parlours'. Day centres usually offer transport to and fro, lunch, activities and medical services such as chiropody etc. 'Pop-ins' are just for tea and a chat.

If you feel energetic, you could join local exercise classes. There are many of these for all age groups. Again, it is not quite like joining a club, because you simply attend, you do not have to commit yourself to anything more than that until you are ready to do so. But it will serve a double purpose of keeping you fit as well as getting you out of the house and into the company of other people. Of course, if you are keen on sport of any kind, joining your local sports club is the ideal way to make new friends.

An alternative to clubs and classes is voluntary work. We are a nation of voluntary workers and there are so many organisations that it is sometimes difficult to choose. In most areas there is a Council of Voluntary Service, which is an umbrella organisation for the whole voluntary sector. You could do worse than have a chat with their Volunteer Co-ordinator who will advise you on where your skills and interests could be best employed. You may be asked to do anything from decorating a flat for a housebound person, to taking care of the cat of an elderly hospitalised lady. If you have a special skill, such as being a trained accountant, a hairdresser, or even a public relations consultant, you may well find a charity that needs an honorary treasurer, an old people's home that would love some free hairdressing for their residents, or an organisation that needs a brochure written or a fundraising campaign masterminded.

At the outset you should tell the Volunteer Co-ordinator or a specific charity exactly how much time you can give them. Be very clear about this – they prefer that, then they know what they can expect from you. If you are working, then you may only be able to help at weekends. If you are not working, do not be tempted to give up all your time to charitable work – you will be worn out, for voluntary work is a bottomless pit and those who run charities admit that they squeeze every last drop of help they can out of people.

One-to-one Relationships

By this I do not just mean dating; there are all sorts of relationships that you can enter into that are on a one-to-one basis. Beware of becoming so involved with one person that your other social life suffers. Some friends can be very demanding and some relationships can become suffocating.

With some people, life can become a ritual series of events. Some always go for a drink with their friends on a Friday night, some always go to bingo on Thursday nights, and so on. Try not to fall into this sort of habit: not only does it become stale after a while, but it also leaves you bereft if it stops.

If you do want to enjoy a one-to-one relationship of a

companionable or intimate nature, there are lots of ways to make contact with other people who want to do the same; of course, they need not have a long-term partnership as an aim unless that is what you want.

Establishing Contacts

Most of the organisations and venues below will advertise in local papers or in specific magazines catering to specific groups, such as single people, widows or senior citizens.

Friendship bureaux: These used to be called marriage bureaux. They are organisations (they may be run from an office or from someone's home) that seek to match up like-minded individuals. Clients fill in a form that asks all sorts of personal questions about lifestyle, hopes, likes and dislikes, hobbies, etc. and it is analysed and 'matched' to a likely candidate for consideration.

Computer dating agencies: These are like the friendship bureaux but use a computer to do the matching.

Video dating agencies: Not for the faint-hearted – registration with such an agency involves sitting in front of a video camera and talking about your ideal mate, your own interest, hopes, fears, etc. Very personal and very damaging to the ego if your looks don't match up to what most of the men want!

Singles clubs: Here we are talking about an actual venue which is specifically for single people. It may be a bar, a restaurant, a disco, or a combination of all three. Single people go there to 'eye up' the possible mates. Fun if you are young, but probably depressing if you are older unless it is a specific 'over-30's' night or similar event.

Event clubs: These can be a good way of meeting people while undertaking an activity that you enjoy, such as going to the theatre or going to a concert.

Dinner clubs: This is also a civilised way of meeting potential soul mates, but without the one-to-one pressure. Groups of single people, usually over the age of 30, meet once a month to have dinner in a restaurant. The organisers prepare a seating plan but there is no pressure to pair off with anyone and it is rather like a convivial dinner party.

Peer group clubs: These are like the above but confined to a membership of people of similar interest or status. For example, a Graduates' Club, or a Managers' Club, or a Teachers' Club, where members of both sexes of similar education and jobs can get together in a social setting.

Holidays: Increasingly popular amongst the over-55 age group. Commercial travel organsiations, such as Saga, organise UK and overseas holidays where single people of both sexes, from the relevant age group, can enjoy the company of others in a supervised holiday programme.

Gay groups: There are lots of gay clubs, pubs and other venues where gay women can meet other gay women. If you have no experience of these you can perhaps first chat to a gay helpline (there are many around the country and they may advertise in gay magazines) and ask some advice as to the best place to go to meet friends.

Contact groups: These are usually for people who have a particular social problem in common or have been through a similar trauma, like divorce or bereavement. The function of these groups is not to provide any romantic possibilities (although that may happen) but to offer contact and support by introducing you to people who have similar problems to yourself. For those who have a problem and feel very isolated, these groups are a valuable way of being re-introduced to society. Details of such groups can be found in libraries, Citizens Advice Bureaux or, sometimes, your doctor's surgery.

Lonely-hearts advertisements: Some thirteen million lonely-hearts or companionship-seeking advertisements appear in the United Kingdom every year, in publications ranging from local newspapers to national magazines and covering all age ranges. It is true that some spectacularly successful relationships have developed through this medium, particularly amongst the elderly. But it is the most 'at risk' medium through which to find a friend. Such advertisements do not tell you very much really and you are risking contact with a stranger who may not turn out to be what you hoped.

SAFETY WHEN YOU GO OUT

You should always be aware of your personal safety when you go out alone.

When meeting someone you know only slightly, suggest that your first meeting is for lunch in a public place and tell a friend where you are going. Do not invite someone into your home until you have come to know them quite well. To avoid putting yourself into a position where you may be trapped, pestered or embarrassed, withold your full address and place of work until you really trust that person.

Most introduction agencies have stringent security regulations. All initial correspondence between potential friends is done through the agency and no addresses are given out until the parties concerned wish to do so. All publications that carry friendship adverts will only publish box numbers and any replies go to the publication first and are then forwarded to the person who has placed the advertisement. When you contact someone who has replied to you, do not give your address. Ring them to arrange a meeting in daylight in a public place. Do not give them a phone number. You will just have to take a chance that they will turn up at the meeting place. Most singles clubs and groups suggest that members just give their first name only until they feel relaxed about the new friends they have made. That way, no one can look up a surname in a phone book and start ringing up and being a nuisance. The safest clubs and groups meet on neutral territory – do not join a group that meets in people's homes.

There are many things you can do, when going out at night, to promote your safety and make it less daunting.

Never, whether during the day or night, walk alone across commons or wasteground, down alleys, quiet or unlit roads, or through pedestrian subways.

Do not expose yourself to risk by waiting alone at bus stops or by entering single or empty carriages on trains. Always sit near the door, try to sit near the driver, guard or conductor, and make a mental note of where the emergency alarm is.

Take only registered cabs, i.e. ones that display licences in the cab and can be telephoned to book your ride. Never accept lifts from strangers and never use 'moonlighting' cabs, no matter how desperate you are. Never tell any cab driver, registered or not, that you live alone. If you arrive at your local station after dark and it is impossible to find a cab, then go to your local police station if it is close by and explain your problem. They would rather let you ring for a cab, or even give you a lift home, than have to deal with any attack that could be made on you on your lonely way home. If there is no police station to hand, go to a public place, such as a garage, and ask to use the phone. Always carry the phone number of a local cab company with you.

When walking alone, particularly at night, always be aware of all the sounds and movements around you. Do not wear a personal stereo headset that blocks out any other noises. Be aware of potential trouble before you walk into it. If, for instance, there is a group of drunks five hundred yards ahead of you, then cross over, or take the next turning to avoid them. Always be sure of your route and walk confidently and purposefully.

If you think that someone is following you, then go into the first public place or lighted house you come to. If the person following you appears to be loitering, then ask the person in charge there or the householder if you can phone the police. No matter how close you are to your home, never let a suspicious person follow you to it so that he – or she – can see you enter an empty house on your own.

Never display anything that may tempt a thief. If possible, put your purse, cheque book and credit cards in an inside coat pocket instead of carrying a handbag. Never put such things in your back trouser pocket – it is very easy to 'pick'.

Do not wear lots of obvious expensive jewellery when you are out. There are other, safer ways of looking glamorous or attractive and lots of gold on display is a powerful temptation to thieves or muggers. Hide necklaces, chains and rings with scarves and gloves.

Always have your car or front door keys ready by the time you need them. You are very vulnerable while you are standing fumbling in your handbag or pockets. Front door keys are best not kept in a handbag anyway, because if your handbag should be stolen you will not be able to enter your home.

If you are really nervous of being out and about or you live in a rough area, invest in a personal alarm. These emit a piercing shriek when activated.

Don't carry it in your handbag, though, keep it in your pocket with your hand on it at all times, ready to press in an emergency.

Be very careful when you withdraw money from street cash dispensers. Never do this at night. If you are elderly, infirm or disabled do not use high street cash dispensers, they are too easy a target for opportunistic thieves.

Don't be predictable. Collect your pension on different days of the week. If you walk home from work, vary your route.

If you are driving alone in a car, do not stop to pick up hitch-hikers; always lock your car doors if you are sitting in a stationary car and do not roll down the window to give a stranger directions. Do not have your handbag in full view on the seat next to you. Thieves have been known to smash car windows and grab the bag, with the driver sitting there.

If you do a lot of driving alone, then invest in a mobile phone so that you can summon help in a breakdown without leaving your car. Always tell the rescue service that you are a woman alone, then they will give you priority.

Keep a torch and a petrol can of fuel in your car and in the winter months carry a warm blanket in case you are snow-bound. A couple of bars of chocolate in the glove compartment is a good idea too!

Always carry good maps of the area you are going to. The better-equipped you are, the more confident you will feel.

If your car breaks down and you have to leave it to get help, take your torch and try to stick to well-lit roads. Do not accept a lift from anyone, even if they seem kindly and unthreatening; ask them, instead, to stop at the next RAC/AA box or garage and ring for help for you.

If you break down on a motorway, you can call for help, using the emergency telephones situated at 1-mile intervals along the carriageway. Arrows on posts on the hard shoulder will point in the direction of the nearest phone. Be ready to give the operator details of your location and a brief description of your car (make, registration number, etc.) so that the rescue patrol can find you quickly. Once you have made your call, go back to your car, but do not sit in it unless the weather is very bad – you are safer sitting on the embankment away from the traffic. If, however, you are too afraid to get out of your car for any reason, you can just stay put and the regular motorway patrols will eventually stop and help you.

As I have already said, being well-equipped does wonders for your confidence. You can take this a step further and attend car maintenance classes – there are some specially designed for women – where you will learn how to deal with minor mechanical problems, change a wheel and so on. Or if you want more help on self-protection, attend a self-defence course. The local police station should be able to advise you on where any such courses may be held. But even the professionals will counsel that, before anything else, when threatened, you should quite simply RUN AND SCREAM AND SHOUT.

Don't be put off going out just because you are alone: the chances of anything happening to you are a great deal less than you probably imagine. And if you follow the advice I have given, you should be as safe as is possible.

Sharing Your Space

This book is meant for women who live alone, so this chapter is not about sharing your living accommodation permanently, but temporarily; perhaps with a pet, perhaps with a guest or a short-term lodger. Any of these things will require some adjustment on your part, because you will have someone or something to think of, apart from yourself, but this may be no bad thing

A period of sharing your home is sometimes healthy, because it teaches you to be more adaptable and stops you from becoming too set in your ways. You ought to be able to cope with a small invasion of your privacy now and then.

It may mean added responsibility, which perhaps is good, if you can cope with it. Remember, a guest of any kind, whether human or pet, is not just someone that is there for your entertainment, it is someone you have to care for.

HAVING FRIENDS AND RELATIVES TO STAY

When you live alone, having friends or relatives to visit

should be a pleasure – something to look forward to – a change from your usual routine. But, as with everything else in life, a little planning and organisation can help to make the pleasure greater because you have anticipated any problems that could arise and dealt with them beforehand, rather than waiting until they happen.

Before the Visit

Find out if there are any special sleeping arrangements to be made: your guest may need a board under the mattress for their bad back, or they may have to have your bedroom because they need to be near the toilet.

Thoroughly clean the place and do as many of the regular household chores before your guest arrives, so that as little as possible has to be done during the visit.

Plan some visits to places of interest, shopping trips or visits to the theatre.

Make sure, when your guest's visit is first arranged, that you decide on a specific start and finish date and time. It does not help you relax and enjoy the company of your guest if you do not know when he or she will arrive and depart.

During the Visit

If you have lived alone for quite a while, you will have your own way of doing things and you may have lost the ability to tolerate the imposition of other people's habits upon you. Lighten up. Yes, the visit is going to be disruptive to your usual pattern of things, but for the duration of the visit you must relax and accept the fact that you will have to clear up after your guests, who may leave the bathroom in a mess and certainly will not know where you put everything in the kitchen. Tell them to make themselves properly at home and, if they are up before you, to make themselves a cup of tea and not feel awkward about it. Show them where everything is, so that if you are out they can look after themselves.

You will probably have to cancel a certain number of your usual social activities while you have a guest staying with you, but do not cancel all of them. If you usually visit an activity club once a week, take your guest with you. If you are a pensioner and usually go to your local day centre or 'pop-in' club, and your guest is of a similar age, ask if they would like to accompany you.

The fact that you have a guest is something to enjoy and make use of, it provides you with an opportunity to do all the things that you have wanted to do but have been unable to do on your own. While you have another pair of hands in the house, you can move heavy pieces of furniture, get your friend to help you pin up those skirts that you have been trying to alter for ages, you could even clean out the guttering as you will have someone to hold the ladder for you! If you have such activities in mind, make sure that your guest knows that he or she is going to do some work during the visit; anyone expecting a complete rest might otherwise be a little taken aback.

I would advise that you do not, if you are working, use up all your holiday time entertaining guests. It is important that you have some time to relax on your own. Looking after the needs of a guest, no matter how comfortable you feel with them, is not a rest. On the other hand, you should not feel that you are too elderly or disabled to have a guest. Organisations such as the Red Cross, the WRVS and the social services will all help you cope by providing extra equipment for a short period, extra meals on wheels or transport.

TEMPORARY LODGERS

You may find it necessary to take in a lodger because you are short of cash, or you may do it to help a friend who has been made homeless. Either way, do not do it unless you have a house or flat that allows for a certain amount of self-containment. Ideally, you should have two bathrooms and be able to provide the person with their own room, in which they can do some cooking if necessary.

You may not be at all happy if you have to share everything that you have been used to having to yourself. You must have some privacy and so must your lodger, and so he should expect to live in his own quarters, not yours.

A woman living alone has to be very careful what sort of lodger she takes in. You may be better off taking in female students or student nurses – it is not against the law to discriminate against men when you are advertising a room for rent. Some private schools that have a lot of foreign pupils advertise for people to give lodging to their pupils during the school holidays. This sort of arrangement could be the perfect solution if you just need to earn some money from your spare room now and then.

There are other kinds of part-time lodgers. For instance, you may find someone who works away from home and would like to rent your spare room during the week but will be going home every weekend. Alternatively, you might consider renting to students from the local college who will be going home during the holidays. It may suit you, if you are out at work all day, to have a night nurse as a lodger. Your paths will only cross for a few hours because, basically, she will sleep during the day while you are out at work and she will be out at work during the night when you are asleep.

If you consider taking lodgers, the main thing is to be certain it is what you want to do and that you have fully researched the pros and cons of the situation.

No matter how well you know the person, do not be casual about the arrangement. Take legal advice and draw up a proper tenancy agreement with carefully defined rules about what the lodger may or may not do, how much the rent is to be and when it is payable, and how long the tenancy period is to last. Otherwise you may have problems making them go if you cannot show that they have contravened a written agreement or that the agreed term of the tenancy has expired. Always give the person a rent book, or give them receipts, and keep a record yourself of all financial transactions. Make sure that the rent you set covers everything that is necessary – light, heat, water, etc. Put a lock on the telephone so that they may only use it with your permission and so that you can make a note of the number dialled and extract it from your itemised bill when it comes in.

Taking in a lodger is fraught with problems, whether it is a friend or a stranger. Friends may think that they can take all sorts of liberties, such as not paying the rent for a week, having other friends in late at night and leaving the place in a mess. Strangers can be even more of a problem because you really do not know anything about them and take them on trust. Ask for references from the applicant's bank manager or employer and always check them.

Before you embark upon the whole business of taking a lodger, get as much information as possible about what is entailed. Talk to your local estate agent: he will tell you about the going rates for rooms in your area and about the pitfalls. It may be that you decide to put the whole business in an estate agent's hands. The advantage of that is that he has all the hassle of collecting rents and drawing up agreements. The disadvantage is that he will take a cut of the rent as a management fee.

Talk to your local tax office too. Rent from a lodger will add to your overall income and you may find that, ultimately, it is not a cost-effective exercise because you may find yourself paying tax for the first time or being pushed up into a higher tax bracket, which eliminates any profit you make from the rent.

Also, if you are in rented accommodation yourself, your lease may not allow you to sub-let. Local authorities usually do allow their tenants to take in lodgers but private landlords may not.

KEEPING PETS

The value of non-human companions is inestimable. It has certainly been proved by the medical profession that stroking an animal lowers human blood pressure (and does a lot for the animal too). But aside from the health benefits, the joy to be derived from pets, the companionship, the interest, and in some cases, the security, are almost beyond words.

My dog makes me laugh, shows me affection constantly, keeps me company, gives me something to cuddle and stroke and keeps me fit. Moreover, when you have a pet, even if it is only a goldfish, it means that you never come home to an empty house.

Keeping pets – providing you take your responsibilities very seriously, genuinely love animals, and look after the pets properly – is marvellous, whether you live alone or with other people.

Choosing the Right Pet

The sort of pet you can keep depends very much on where you live, whether you work or are out all day, and how much money you have. Any dog really should live in a house with a garden, and have an accompanied walk every day, with some time off the leash during which to run around. It will cost at least £1 a day to feed, needs some companionship during the day, and all sorts of other commitments from you which, on consideration, you may not be prepared to make. A cat is less demanding (it does not need to be taken for walks for a start) and a fish even less so (although some expensive tropical fish need careful temperature control and special food).

Whatever pet you choose you will also have to buy a number of accessories – leads, collars, balls, beds, cages, bells, tanks and so on. As I mentioned in the chapter on managing money, you can take out a special pet health insurance to help you cope with all the vets' bills, which you will undoubtedly have.

You may live in a place where pets that run around, like cats and dogs, are not allowed. Some councils are still strict about allowing tenants to keep certain pets, and most sheltered accommodation complexes, whether rented or private, are also strict about keeping pets.

You must be realistic about your age and mobility too. It is not fair to keep a dog if you are unable to take it for walks – even a small lap dog. If you cannot manage to clean your house or flat every day, you should not keep six cats either, because the place will smell appalling very quickly.

You must think about the time you have available to spend with an animal. If all the time you can spare is literally five minutes in the morning before you go to work and a couple of hours in the evening when you come home, then you would probably be better off with a caged animal, such as a hamster or a bird. No pet should be ignored. All pets need food, clean bedding, decent living conditions and amusement. Even birds need toys and fish must have some plants and rocks to swim around.

Of course, keeping a pet – any pet – means that you cannot go on holiday without making arrangements for someone else to look after it. I have never been able to put my dog in kennels when I go away. I either leave her with someone that she likes and trusts, or ask someone to stay at my house and look after her. I know many other dog and cat owners who feel the same.

If, in the end, you decide to keep a pet, you must choose it very carefully. Age Concern run an advisory service whereby they match pets up to elderly people. The RSPCA, PDSA, or any of the other animal organisations that exist will be able to advise you about particular pets that you may be interested in keeping. Your local vet will also advise you and will probably have leaflets on pet care that have been published by the various pet food manufacturers.

Health and Pets

Any pet will incur veterinary bills. There will be annual innoculations, medicines for various ailments, like worms and fleas, and perhaps various operations like spaying or neutering, apart from emergency fees. It can be expensive.

There are certain hazards to human health as well as benefits from animals. Even the cleanest of dogs can pick up worms and one of these – toxicara canis – can cause blindness in humans if they come into contact with it. Therefore all dog's faeces in the garden should be cleared up daily and disposed of. Cats also can transmit diseases through their waste products, so you should be especially careful when handling litter trays. The cleanest of dogs and cats can pick up fleas, particularly if dogs go rabbiting in the woods when you let them off the leash. One flea can lay hundreds of eggs, which can infest your carpets and furniture in no time, especially if you have central heating. There are sprays, powders and shampoos for sale, of course, as well as flea collars, anti-flea drops which are applied to the animal's skin once a month and anti-flea tablets/powders you mix into the animal's food which effectively stop fleas from laying eggs.

Birds can transmit the disease psittacosis to humans, so

you should never 'kiss' a budgie, as some people often do. Mice, rats, hamsters, gerbils, guinea pigs and rabbits can bite clean through your finger if they feel like it.

Problems with Pets

Some of the other negative aspects of keeping pets are the mess that they make. Dogs and cats shed hairs and trail mud through clean houses. Puppies will defecate and urinate on the floor until they are house-trained (which is quite a lengthy and trying process) and when they are teething, they may chew skirting boards, the legs of your furniture and any loose objects they can reach while you are out. Some dogs howl if they are left alone in the house and puppies will initially whine at night. Cats love to scratch the furniture (even if they have a scratching post) and most of them like to climb the curtains.

Any kind of rodent tends to be a nocturnal creature and may well keep you awake at night, scampering about its cage. Singing canaries and talking birds may drive you to distraction with their constant noise.

Despite the problems, though, I would not personally be without a pet. Many of my friends feel the same way too. A widowed neighbour of mine found that acquiring a dog helped her to overcome the loss of her husband; a busy career woman of my acquaintance says 'Money couldn't buy the kind of welcome that I get from my cats when I get home at night'.

Animal Intruders

While your pets may be lovely, other people's pets, particularly cats that dig up your garden and defecate over it, are not.

Any animal that is the property of another person is protected under the Protection of Animals Act 1911, which makes it an offence to cause undue suffering to a domestic animal. So, much as you would like to shoot or poison next door's cat, you should not even throw anything at it – except water. You can deter cats and dogs by using substances which give off smells that they find unpleasant. These preparations are sold at garden centres, and come in either spray, pellet, wax or powder form for application to plants, or to the ground.

Beware, however: if you have pets of your own, or your garden is visited by other people's pets, or you like to encourage birds to feed in your garden, do not put bait down to kill slugs, or you will poison the animal or birdlife that you want to encourage.

WILDLIFE

If, after a great deal of thought, you feel that your busy lifestyle prohibits you from keeping a pet, or you cannot cope with the responsibilities, then you can always encourage the local wildlife to share your garden and indulge your love of animals in that way.

Putting up a bird table where you can easily see it from your living room and keeping it well stocked, should provide you with hours of pleasure watching birds coming and going. If you are lucky you may also attract some squirrels to the bird table. A nesting box, or two, in shady places, might attract small birds when they start their families. You could even invest in a bat-box, if you know that there are bats locally. Planting certain kinds of plants in your garden, such as buddleia bushes, will attract butterflies. Having a garden pond may attract frogs or toads.

The RSPCA publish many leaflets on encouraging wildlife activity in your garden. Their advice is sound and shows you how to encourage wildlife without encouraging pests.

Unwanted Pests

Most of the wildlife in your garden is harmless, possibly slightly destructive to lawns or plants, but certainly not likely to attack humans, unless severely provoked.

Your local Environmental Health department may be empowered to deal with foxes, rats, mice, rabbits, pigeons, starlings, feral cats and wasps' nests. They charge a fee for some activities but not for others. It varies from council to council. They will not necessarily exterminate them but may encourage them to move on and offer advice on how to protect your garden against them. Many local councils no longer offer this service, however, and will refer you to private pest control firms. The local authority, Cats' Protection League or RSPCA can help advise you on feral cats. If you think you have foxes, or even badgers, do not leave bits of food about or rubbish in easy-to-get-to plastic bags.

Moles, hedgehogs and badgers, although delightful to watch, can be a nuisance, but they are basically harmless. Hedgehogs will benefit your garden by eating all the slugs. You cannot do anything about badgers, as they are protected by law, you will just have to wait for them to move on. You could contact the local branch of the RSPCA to ask their advice. Moles are supposed to be deterred by the smell of any plant from the onion family – onion, garlic or leek. Plant these in between your prize roses, or sink slates or paving stones at intervals along your flower beds to stop moles burrowing. Another method of deterring them is to plant empty glass bottles along the edge of flower beds, with the necks exposed. The noise made when the wind blows across the top of the bottle necks is supposed to unnerve moles, who have very sensitive hearing. The RSPCA publishes some very useful booklets about dealing with moles, foxes, badgers and hedgehogs.

If you have a larger fishpond, you may even attract herons, kingfishers and seagulls. You may appreciate seeing them but they are expert at taking fish. You can stop this from happening by putting a wire mesh over the pond, just under the water.

Infestations of any kind can be dealt with the your local Environmental Health department (or a private firm – look in the Yellow Pages) for a modest fee.

Conclusion

*T*here are so many practical elements to consider when you take on the responsibility of running your own home – from finances to food, health to entertainment. Hopefully, I have covered all the important practical elements in this book, so that you have a useful guide to help you sort out all those situations you may never have encountered before. When you are facing something unknown, especially if it's a problem – however minor – it is reassuring to know that someone else has been there before and found straightforward and workable solutions.

Another important element which I hope I have communicated is how positive an experience living alone can be – and indeed should be. Some of you will have chosen to live alone, others may have felt forced into it through change of circumstances. Each of you will have a different attitude to your situation. But by concentrating on the positive and working to eliminate, or at least minimize, any negative aspects you come across, you really can find it a rewarding experience.

Index of Useful Names and Addresses

Age Concern   Astral House, 1268 London Road, London SW16 4ER *Advice and practical help for the elderly.*

Alcoholics Anonymous   PO Box 1, Stonebow House, Stonebow, York YO1 2NJ *Help and support for anyone with a drink problem.*

Association of British Insurers   51 Gresham Street, London EC2V 7HQ *Advice on insurance and home security.*

British Red Cross Society   9 Grosvenor Crescent, London SW1X 7EJ *Sources of aid and temporary appliances for the elderly and disabled.*

The Building Societies Association   3 Savile Row, London W1X 1AF *General information about home buying and borrowing money.*

Citizens Advice Bureau (National Association of) 115–123 Pentonville Road, London N1 9LZ *Practical advice and help across a wide range of legal and domestic problems.*

Consumers Association   2 Marylebone Road, London NW1 4DF *Advice and literature on consumer matters.*

Counsel and Care (for the Elderly)   Tyman House, Lower Ground Floor, 16 Bonny Street, Camden, London NW1 9PG *Advice and help for the elderly.*

Cruse   Cruse House, 126 Sheen Road, Richmond, Surrey TW9 1UR *Advice, help and publications for the widowed.*

DAERA (Disability Alliance Educational & Research Association)   Universal House, 88–94 Wentworth Street, London E1 7SA *Information and advice on social security benefits, training and employment opportunities for disabled people.*

DGAA - Homelife (Formerly the Distressed Gentlefolks Aid Association)   Vicarage Gate House, Vicarage Gate, Kensington, London W8 4AQ *Practical and financial help for retired professional people.*

Help the Aged   St James Walk, London EC1R 0BE *Advice and help for the elderly.*

Holiday Care Service   2 Old Bank Chambers, Station Road, Horley, Surrey RH6 9HW *Advice on holidays for those with special needs.*

Law Centres Federation   Duchess House, 18–19 Warren Street, London W1P 5DB *List of local centres where free legal advice is given.*

The Law Society of England and Wales   113 Chancery Lane, London WC2A 1PL *Advice on complaints against the legal profession.*

The Law Society of Northern Ireland   98 Victoria Street,

Belfast BT1 3JZ *Advice on complaints against the legal profession.*
The Law Society of Scotland 26 Drumsheugh Gardens, Edinburgh EH3 7YR *Advice on complaints against the legal profession.*
MIND (National Association for Mental Health) 15–19 Broadway, London E15 4BQ *Advice and help for the mentally ill.*
National Association of Victim Support Schemes Cranmer House, 29 Brixton Road, London SW9 6DZ *Help and advice for the victims of crime.*
National Association of Widows 54–57 Allison Street, Digbeth, Birmingham B5 5TH *Advice for the widowed.*
National Council for the Divorced and Separated 8 South Knighton Road, Leicester LE2 3LN *Advice for the divorced and separated.*
RELATE (formerly the National Marriage Guidance Council) Herbert Gray College, Little Church Street, Rugby, Warwicks CV21 3AP *Advice and help with any personal relationship and literature on coping alone.*
RELEASE 388 Old Street, London EC1V 9LT *Advice on legal, criminal and drug-related problems.*
RoSPA (Royal Society for the Prevention of Accidents) The Safety Centre, 353 Bristol Road, Birmingham B5 7ST *Advice on accident prevention in the home.*
RSPCA (Royal Society for the Prevention of Cruelty to Animals) The Causeway, Horsham, West Sussex RH12 1HG *Advice about pets and practical help with wildlife.*
The Salvation Army 101 Queen Victoria Street, London EC4P 4EP *Practical support and centres for the lonely.*
WRVS (Womens Royal Voluntary Service) 234–244 Stockwell Road, London SW9 9SP *Practical help for the lonely, housebound and elderly. Also national organisation seeking volunteer workers.*

Index